Letting Go

Release Your Suffering

SUZHEN LIU

BALBOA.PRESS

A DIVISION OF HAY HOUSE

Balboa Press books may be ordered through booksellers or by contacting:

Balboa Press
A Division of Hay House
1663 Liberty Drive
Bloomington, IN 47403
www.balboapress.com
844-682-1282

Print information available on the last page.

ISBN: 978-1-9822-5800-9 (sc)
ISBN: 978-1-9822-5799-6 (hc)
ISBN: 978-1-9822-5798-9 (e)

Library of Congress Control Number: 2020921619

Balboa Press rev. date: 12/15/2020

How it all came about

Enlightened teachers are hard to come by and it is even more rare that someone can give us concrete and pragmatic instructions on how to follow suit. Suzhen Liu is a gem from Taiwan who has accomplished both of these feats. We are delighted to introduce her treasure from the East, Letting Go—Release Your Suffering, to the West.

Suzanne Yang is her mentee and has worked for years at Suzhen Liu's side practicing and teaching her healing methods. At a time of great personal struggle, Suzanne effectively used Letting Go—Release Your Suffering for her own healing. It was then that she decided that this book needed to be shared with the Western world and I helped her to get it published.

I met Suzanne in a spiritual community that soon after closed down due to some internal quarrels between the owner of the group and its administrators. Suzanne and I decided that we are now called to start a community of our own and couldn't have found a better start than sharing Suzhen Liu's spiritual wisdom and effective healing methods. Letting Go—Release Your Suffering will change your life. It has transformed ours!

The Chinese original of Letting Go—Release your Suffering was released in 2018 by ECUS Publishing House in Taiwan as "The Work "當下的釋放"". This book is a collection of seminar notes that T. Y. Lee put together. He is a senior counselor with a master's degree from National Taiwan University and has worked with Suzhen Liu for over twenty years. We thank him for writing the introduction and for providing many other helpful suggestions.

We thank ECUS Publishing House for granting us the rights to publish this book. Corinne Habib provided tireless editing work and we also thank Juhi Dhawan and Eric Crowley for their valuable feedback.

Christian M. Wiese
Author of The Way of the Meister

CONTENTS

INTRODUCTION BY T. Y. LEE

The first time people hear of The Letting Go Method, the question that often arises is, "How can it be that you can resolve your deep rooted issues just by saying a few sentences?" Yet, it is true! As long as you are willing to learn The Method, experience it, and invoke its inner healing power and wisdom, you will be surprised to discover that we can activate such a strong healing power within us.

Suzhen Liu discovered The Letting Go Method by accident. Suzhen had been practicing Qigong for a while. She had become very efficient in healing herself using different Qigong techniques. One day, however, when she tried to heal her leg pain, no matter how much she tried, she just couldn't make the pain go away. She said to herself, "Let go of this pain energy." Surprisingly, after she finished this sentence, she burst into tears and the image of being punished by her father when she was a little girl surfaced. Soon the pain in her leg went away. That's how she discovered The Letting Go Method.

This method ignites mental and physical changes in people who practice it. One of my students told me, "You looked like an old man 10 years ago when I attended the seminar led by you, but now you look much younger!" The changes that happened to me were brought about by The Letting Go Method. It has loosened up the pain and stuck energy within me. It has a very strong purification power.

Letting Go of Mental Wounds

Why does The Letting Go Method have such a strong power? This is because there is energy in all the words and sentences we speak. If you can say the right sentences for example, you can let go of the sad energy you have been carrying around. The energy of the right sentence can help us clear out the entangled energy that we have been stuck with.

"What is your mindset when you are in pain?", Master Suzhen Liu invited us to inquire. "Do you try your best to get rid of this sadness, anger or grief? Whenever you are trying to get rid of your pain, you are fighting with it. Our pain is created by our mindset. Trying to get rid of the pain is equivalent to fighting one mindset with another. You then feel conflicted and get stuck. When you are paying attention to your pain, you will focus your energy on your attentiveness and all the conflicts and struggles will stop. When you are paying attention to your pain, your pain starts a transformation." This is the key element of The Letting Go Method.

We relax ourselves to observe the changes in us after saying the Letting Go Sentences out loud. We are quiet and observe the changes in our body, mind and energy. When we observe, we are in a state of paying attention. At this moment, we don't have "want" or "don't want" on our mind. When we observe ourselves silently, the stuck and frozen energy starts moving again. This is the mechanism behind The Letting Go Method. When our mind stops fighting and intervening with the pain, the energy in our body moves smoothly. What used to bother us transforms into the nutrition nurturing our evolution.

Transforming Your Suffering, Transforming Your Destiny

You can apply The Letting Go Method mentally and physically. For example, when your body doesn't feel well, when you are in a negative mood, when you suffer from insomnia or have an eating disorder. It's especially effective for healing mental wounds. For example, your mom may have said to you when you were a little child, "If you don't behave, I will get rid of you!" You felt the threat of being abandoned. You also concluded that your mom didn't love you and you said to yourself, "I am not important." All these feelings enhance each other. Very soon you have an overwhelming feeling of abandonment.

When mothers say those things to their children, a child can feel hurt, wronged and depressed. A little child doesn't know how to express these feelings and emotions. This hurt becomes an unfinished emotion, an unfinished energy. Nature has a power to finish whatever is unfinished. After we feel hurt, to prevent us from being hurt again, our mind will try to get rid of the feeling of being hurt. If you feel abandoned, you will seek recognition. If you feel unloved, you will look for love. If you never know how to let go of these emotions, you may spend your whole life with this pain.

In other words, when we experience these hurts, these pain bodies become part of our world. The Letting Go Method loosens the grip between your life and these hurts. This method will change your destiny and change your world! The power of letting go enables you to finish with these unloved emotions. It frees you of your hurts and completes these endless loops you were caught in.

Let Flow What's Frozen; Free Yourself by Forgiving

Any hurt can result in frozen energy. Whenever we let go of this hurt, we initiate the flow of this frozen energy. After the frozen energy flows naturally, we can accept what happened and forgive the person who hurt us. However, if we try to forgive mentally, forgiveness won't happen. Forgiveness is a full body experience. You may tell yourself, "He didn't mean it. He treated me so badly because he was hurt himself." Yet, you will very often feel conflicted if you merely try to convince yourself to forgive.

You can only forgive people after you let the frozen energy flow and heal the hurt. The Letting Go Method loosens up the entangled energy and helps find closure from the episode when you got hurt. After we resolve the feeling of being hurt, we won't react to our current life situation from a wounded place. Instead, we discover the beauty of this present moment and all of the implicit possibilities. We are free!

Awareness and Concentration

Once you finish your Letting Go Sentence, pay attention to yourself. Paying attention is often confused with concentration. When you are watching a movie, or when you try to solve a complex equation, you devote yourself so much to the activity that you cannot notice anything else. This is concentration. Concentration is exclusive. When you concentrate on something, you cannot notice anything else. Paying attention is different. When you pay attention, you are open. Your energy is not occupied by anything else. You are relaxed. The attention we need to learn in The Letting Go Method is open and all inclusive.

Digging into Your Deep Belief Sets

We come to all sorts of conclusions when we feel hurt. For example, we may conclude that "I am not important" and then we use this conclusion to interpret our life and our relationships with others with this mindset. We let the hurts we experienced in the past form the reality of our world, our self, and our relationships.

By applying The Letting Go Method, the belief sets we have about our own life, our money, and our health surface and give us the opportunities to loosen up the presumptions that we have created for our life.

We are so used to repressing ourselves. We don't allow ourselves to cry, not to mention, to get angry. Crying is an important part in The Letting Go Method. Crying allows energy to flow. When you cry, your breath changes, your tears stream down and they bring out the accumulated toxins of heavy metals, adrenaline, and hormones.

There are tears and sound when you cry. Please allow yourself to cry with sound. When you cry with sound, your pain will be released from the area of the diaphragm. Please allow yourself to cry totally. If you only cry with tears and without sound, you are only using your head to cry, and you cannot experience total release. If you are not used to weeping out loud, you can just pretend to cry. Sometimes you will burst into tears when you pretend to cry.

People who cannot cry carry more pain than people who are able to cry. For these people this energy is so stuck that they become numb. When you are not able to feel pain, you cannot feel joy either. So, we have to learn to be present with our pain. When the painful energy is able to flow, it's much easier for us to feel happy and peaceful.

Venting versus Letting Go

Venting is different than letting go. When you vent, you vent with your stories. The Letting Go Method is different. When you practice The Letting Go Method to deal with your emotions, you detach from your storylines. So, your crying will come to an end more quickly. On the other hand, if you use venting to deal with your emotions, there seems to be no end to your crying and complaints.

When you practice The Letting Go Method, you are present. Being present with your practice means you don't have any hopes or fears. You don't wish things to be otherwise and neither are you afraid of what is to come. In contrast, when you vent, you indulge yourself in your storyline. There is fear, hope, want and don't want. You indulge yourself with demands such as, "How can he treat me like this? I wish he had treated me differently!"

When you are practicing The Letting Go Method, you are in the present moment. When you vent, you live in your head, in the future and in the past. If you keep saying, "That person treats me badly! Poor me!", you are venting. If you are present with your emotions, you are practicing The Letting Go Method. The pain will end because you detach yourself from your pain.

The Six Steps of The Letting Go Method

1. You are aware of your worries and obstacles.

2. You are aware that if you repeat your old patterns, you will hurt yourself and others. So, stop these patterns.

3. You understand that if you want to run away or get rid of these negative emotions you will be creating conflicts within yourself and prolong your own suffering. Therefore, you are willing to face these negative emotions.

4. When you first connect with this uneasiness, some emotional baggage will surface. You can experiment with some Letting Go Sentences and say them aloud. Even if they cannot exactly describe how you feel, it's ok. Some more appropriate sentences may surface later.

5. As you stay present, the layers of your frozen emotions will show up layer by layer.

6. New Letting Go Sentences will surface as we continue the practice. As we let go, layer by layer, of our frozen emotions, we will understand ourselves and have new insights.

The Factors

The process of letting go is the process of knowing yourself. There are a lot of factors that may influence how it turns out. For example, if you can't find the corresponding Letting Go Sentences; if you are used to repressing yourself; if you feel suspicious about The Letting Go Method; if you want to get rid of your negative emotions when you practice The Letting Go Method; how much you know and understand yourself—these are all possible factors. The more you know yourself, the easier it will be for you to find the corresponding Letting Go Sentences. The stiller you are, the easier it will be for you to let go the layers of your frozen energy and the deeper you can go into yourself. You won't be trapped in your emotions easily or run away from them.

The Letting Go Method can untie your physical and mental knots and guide you toward yourself. When you follow the leads of this book, and try to understand yourself step by step, you will realize it is your thinking patterns and attitudes that create your pain. For example, your expectations toward your family, or seeking recognition from your partner, create all the tensions between you. If you can keep letting go of the frozen energy and finally see the person who creates all these issues, you will be free!

Time to apply The Letting Go Method

1. For eyes:

If you spend a lot of time with your smartphone or your computer, and you feel that your eyes get tired or strained, you should give yourself some time away from the screen. You can also practice The Letting Go Method to release the negative energy trapped in your eyes. You can in fact feel hot air getting released from your eyes. You only need to practice this for a few minutes. Most of the time the discomfort will stop right away.

If you witness something horrifying, you can apply The Letting Go Method to help release the tumultuous energy. It will calm you down and prevent the buildup of any damaging after effects. For example, if you witness a car accident, it often happens that your mind will be haunted with these disturbing images. You can practice The Letting Go Method at this moment to release the negative energy that you were exposed to and release the horrifying energy that you feel. Whenever you witness anything unpleasant, you can apply this method to release the haunting effect it has on you. You can also apply the same method to whatever disaster or horror you are exposed to on TV. Often we feel resistant to what we've seen and our resistance creates even more suffering for us. The presence and attention we carry out while practicing this method helps us to undo this resistance. It helps us to unlock the frozen energy and enables us to let the energy flow away. Sometimes our discomfort just comes from receiving this negative energy. Sometimes these horrific images trigger our own painful memories. When you pay attention and are present, the past memory will often resurface and you can then release the past event. You can feel more relaxed after these practices.

2. For ears:

You can let go of the negative energy after you hear someone's troublesome story, after a fight, or after having being scolded. When we have to stay in a noisy or in a conflict ridden environment, we will accumulate the resistance and negative energy in our ears. One of my students suffered from long term earache. She had all sorts of different tests done but the doctors couldn't find a cause. When I asked her to release the earache, she felt a lot of hot air release from her ears and images of her sister surfaced. It turned out that they had a strained relationship for a long time. Her sister was often hostile to her and said nasty things to her. She felt pain after these fights but felt that there was nothing that she could do about it. In fact, she wished that she didn't have this sister. After practicing The Method, she realized that all the negative emotions had accumulated in her ears. She also knew she had to face and repair their relationship. Magically, at that moment, her earaches just disappeared.

3. Contaminated food:

You can practice The Letting Go Method after you have consumed contaminated food. You can release the negative energy that your body has absorbed.

4. Bad air:

If you breathe in smoke or paint fumes and feel uncomfortable, you can release the negative energy you inhaled into your lungs with the help of The Method.

5. Conflict ridden exposure:

If you feel uncomfortable after visiting heavy energy locations such as hospitals or funeral homes, you can release the negative energy that you have absorbed. Sometimes we feel heavy after speaking to depressed people. We can let go of the negative energy that we have received.

6. Worry and fear:

For example, someone always felt uneasy at night. When he let go of the uneasy energy he experienced at night, images resurfaced of his drunken father returning home late and fighting with his mom. He could then release the fear and energy of feeling helpless. Our worries and fears are mostly from our past memories. Releasing these wounded memories free us from these experienced traumas.

We can also practice The Letting Go Method to release our other fears and can manage to know ourselves better. For example, we can let go of the fear of authority, the fear of being late, the fear of being in the limelight, the fear to express different opinions, or the fear of rejecting others or being rejected.

7. TV, movies, dramas, news:

When we are triggered by TV, movies, dramas, or news often there lie our unhealed wounds. Pay attention to your emotion. You can know yourself better when you practice this method and unlock your obstacles. Some people like to use TV viewing in order to vent. However, if you are not present with yourself and don't know why you are crying, your crying is just venting. You will cry again when similar scenarios happen. Be present when you are triggered, you will then understand and end this trauma, and your obstacle will be released. Afterwards, you will then respond very differently when you watch similar dramas.

8. When you cannot fall asleep:

If your being awake is not being caused by some physical reason, you can let go of the energy that is keeping you up. Some old traumas or a more recent annoyance may surface. The reasons for insomnia can be complicated. In addition to old injuries, it can be related to your compulsive thinking patterns. Observing yourself and using The Letting Go Method may help you release the thinking patterns that can help free you from these diseases.

9. Indecisions:

When you don't know how to make a decision, you can let go of the energy of indecision. Indecision can be very torturing. People around you will be influenced too.

When you let go of the energy of indecision, the regretful energy of prior wrong decisions may surface which make you too scared to make a decision now. So, the key is not about choosing A or B, but to understand the worries beneath. Or you can try to release the worries beneath each decision as a way to better know yourself.

10. When things don't go your way:

You can release the energy of disappointment or frustration and discover your underlying expectations.

11. When you want to make demands or blame someone for your worries:

Pause and feel your worries. Let go of your worries and express your concerns when you feel more relaxed.

In a word, just practice The Letting Go Method whenever worries or unease arise within you. You can always connect with yourself and others much better when you are practicing this method.

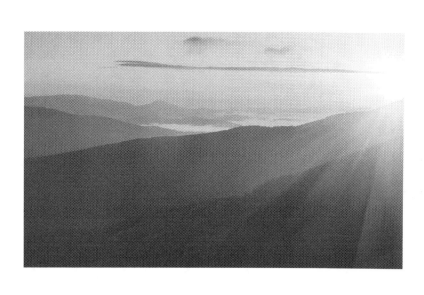

CHAPTER 1

Why Don't You Love Me After I Have Done So Much for You?

The lives of most people are like broken records. They live under the influence of their memories. They repeat their past dramas and they draw the people around them into this play. We cannot really build real relationships with anyone unless we can heal our old wounds. Otherwise, we just repeat the old dramas with someone new.

The real happiness in a relationship doesn't come from living "happily ever after." The real happiness in a relationship comes after both have been through a lot together and still decide to hold each other's hand. We gain our wisdom and strength after we have been through life's storms. We live in peace and love after these episodes.

When a couple can still be together after having gone through a lot, it shows that they both have learned something. When both are learning from their life spent

1

together—either through repressing or transcending—they are looking at life as it is steadily changing and no longer look at life the way it used to be. They no longer demand life to happen according to their expectations. Once both can look at life with an open heart, real happiness starts flowing into their relationship. When you can embrace what life brings your way there is no more suffering. It is the most challenging thing to learn from a relationship. We are influenced by every interaction our partner shares with us.

A mother once told me, "My son is looking for a job now and he has a lot of stress. One day he came home and said to me, 'I know you love me but you are overshadowing me. You raised me like a loser!' I felt so sad after he said that to me. I was not into awareness at that time so I could only react to what he said. I felt angry, so I told him, 'How dare you say that to me after I've dedicated my whole life to you?' And then we had a big fight."

We always take action in relationships according to our own motivation. Perhaps we take action out of fear. We fear that the other person will leave us. So, we devote ourselves to him to keep him around. We also expect things to go as planned even though it may not happen this way. As a matter of fact, when we take action out of fear, we cannot really connect with the other. What we have done may not meet the other person's needs and pressure him even more. Try to understand your motivation first. Then you won't have resentment towards the other. It's very important to know your motivation so you won't be disappointed when things don't go according to plan.

To have good relationships, the most important thing is to observe and to know ourselves. However, most of us do it the other way around. We do our best to please others, to show our love without knowing our own motivation. When we have no idea what we are doing, when we have no idea who we are—we often do things out of our own drama. We cannot really connect with someone and give them what they need.

Why do we suffer so much in our relationships? It's very obvious that we love each other very much but why do we feel frustrated and angry at times? It's because we are under the influence of "should" and of our own thinking. In other words, our relationships are ruled by our minds. For example, most people have expectations about how mothers should interact with their children, or how children should interact with their mothers, or how a husband should behave, or what a wife should do. Once we interact with a person's "should" or thinking, it is inevitable that we will feel disappointed when the other person doesn't behave according to our expectations. We need to communicate with our partner on how to change the way we interact with each other or frustration and anger will build. Once we accumulate a lot of frustration and anger, it's inevitable that our relationship will deteriorate.

It's challenging to have a good relationship. We need to learn how to do it. We can only learn to love each other by understanding each other. When we can understand someone, we will be able to love them. When we can understand the other, we can accept his behavior. We won't be triggered by his words or behavior.

To understand each other, we need to put down our expectations, or know what kind of expectations we have towards our partners and interactions. Once we can see clearly how often we act under the influence of "should" and our thinking, we can then slowly dismantle these minefields.

We cannot consciously accept others. We can only accept others by understanding them. To understand them is to love them. It won't work when we force ourselves to accept them since we then act according to our mind and not reality. When you tolerate the other only from a mind level, even if you control yourself not to lose your temper at that special moment, you will lose it one day soon.

Even if you want to love the other, you cannot make it if you are under the control of your mind. Love can only succeed when you understand your own suffering and thinking patterns.

It is our nature to want to be loved because we need to belong and to feel secure. However, when we want to be loved, we are looking from outside, and the relationship is controlled by others. Under these circumstances, even if we experience fleeting happiness, we cannot truly feel happy.

Is it because we are not doing it right, or not working hard enough? Of course not. We don't feel happy because we "think" we need to work hard in order to feel happy. Or, we think we need to do something to own happiness, so we keep looking for it outside, and forget to look within. We are conditioned by our "thinking." We only feel frustrated and painful after we exert a lot of effort, and happiness eludes us.

Actually, the outside cannot give you happiness. You can only find your happiness when love arises in your heart. When we turn within, that is, when we get to the source where our issues originate and our thoughts arise, we are bound to discover big treasures. We will find all of our injuries within—the resentment, anger, frustration, the feeling of having been wronged and despair. Only when we understand them, peace arises in our heart. It is then when we feel harmonious and happy.

You don't have to work hard to feel happy. You feel happy by understanding, by having clarity and insights. Apply the same mindfulness method to all your daily interactions. Follow this energy and naturally your life will be filled with love.

To understand yourself, I invite you to learn healing through The Letting Go Method.

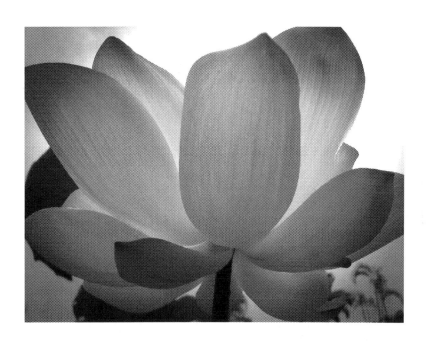

CHAPTER 2

Release Your Suffering: Start with Observing Your Inner Self

When I was in my twenties, several family members passed away. First, it was my father. I took care of him when he was in the hospital in southern Taiwan. He passed away after being sick for a while. I arranged his funeral and everything that needed to be taken care of. Then my sister passed away, followed shortly by my mother. In less than 3 months, I lost three family members. I was in total chaos and suffered incredibly. I had originally planned to have a physical check-up done before these tragedies, but then I lost interest in seeing the doctor altogether.

When I finally got the check-up done, the doctor said that I had some abnormal cells. It was not easy to get medical information 30 years ago. I didn't know what abnormal cells were but the doctors said that I could die soon. It was a terrible period of time for me. Not only did I lose three family members, the doctor also told me that I might die in one month. This triggered a dramatic change in my life. It took me 6 days and 5 nights. After that, I felt that I was finally alive!

Why Was I Always Thinking of Someone Else?

After the doctor's appointment, and the prognosis about my life, I went home. The first thought I had was, "What's the big deal about death? There is not so much to live for anyway!" This wasn't true. It was a thought after all. When you really face death, all the attachments to life will show up.

I thought that I was not scared of death. However, the moment I really faced the possibility of death, I had that intense feeling that my life was going to end soon. This was something that I had never experienced before. So, I started crying, crying desperately; crying for a very long time but I had no idea what I was crying about. Maybe I cried because I was dying. I didn't know. I had never cried like this before.

When I was crying, thoughts popped up nonstop. "What's going to happen to my son if I die?" "What's going to happen to my money if I die?" "What's going to happen to my boyfriend if I die?" I cried and cried, and cried. I cried from afternoon to night. When I was lost in tears, suddenly a question hit me, "Why am I only thinking of other people when I am going to die?"

I was confused. I was totally confused. Why was I only thinking of others when I was going to die? Why didn't I think of myself?

Don't Waste Your Life on Things

Suddenly, I calmed down. Suddenly, I saw my life. What occupied my life? Every day I spent time worrying about my son, about his studies and his future. Every day I was thinking about my dates with my boyfriend. Every day I was thinking about how much money I had.

It was at that special moment when I realized, being just in my twenties, that I lived with these thoughts, lived with these attachments; that I always wanted more, always wanted to be better, always wanted to accumulate. But they were not making me happy. To the contrary, they made me scared of losing what I had.

Should we live our life like this? I was shocked! It wasn't until that unique moment that I realized that I had never really lived my life! I was a dead woman walking! After I reached these realizations I started crying again. How could that be? A lot of things came to the surface. I didn't know what to do and just let them flow. I had never followed any gurus. I realized then that my sufferings are my guru.

On the sixth day, I cried again. This crying was very fierce, deep, and painful! It was totally different than the crying

9

of the prior 5 days. Because this time I saw all the people leading their life this same way—my son, my brothers, my family. Everyone lives in this delusional world. Everyone lives under the influence of their thoughts. Everyone lives with competition. No one really lives their life!

For six straight days, I had cried nonstop. However, I didn't feel tired. On the contrary, I felt energized. I didn't really do anything in these six days. I just saw clearly how I had lived my life in the past two decades. I saw how I had accumulated this pain unconsciously. It was only at the time when I was facing death that I finally saw how I had lived my life.

Reborn

After all those days of crying I became a different person. The way I looked at life was transformed. Everything changed from that moment on. It is not that I have had a free, glamorous life since that day. I still experienced a lot of pain and suffering. However, I suddenly understood that these are all learning opportunities. I have embraced everything coming into my life! My temper has also changed completely.

When you try to understand the meaning beneath your suffering, your life becomes different! It's a beautiful thing to learn about our life! It's a beautiful thing to understand our life! Don't be scared to face yourself!

This understanding has to come from our own willingness to learn and know ourselves. We can't force ourselves to do things like this. I didn't talk to anyone in those six days. No one taught me anything. It's very simple and easy to discover yourself when you are willing to face yourself!

The Power of Being Present

When I was young, I felt that my life was meaningless! Whatever I did, I felt lonely even when I spent my time with many people.

In my twenty years of life, I was not happy. I wanted a lot of stuff, however, when I finally got it, I was not really happy either. My boyfriend once bought me a diamond. When I put it on, I was still not happy. I was not happy and I didn't know how to be happy until I discovered The Letting Go Method. After this, I had a totally different feeling about life. Life has become fresh, beautiful, and different! It's almost like I have a totally different heart than before! I am finally alive! No guru, no spiritual practice, no meditation. All you need is simply to face yourself, no matter if it is ugly or embarrassing! Just be present with yourself!

You need to be present with yourself to see your truth, the absolute reality of yourself. When we are able to see our absolute absolute reality—the power, strength, and wisdom will emerge.

Releasing Your Inner Suffering Patterns

In 1999, I went to help people impacted by the big earthquake in central Taiwan. I felt heartbroken when I saw their collapsed houses. Every broken house represented a broken family. When my eyes locked with a survivor's eyes, the air froze. I could never forget those eyes. Those eyes revealed the pain of losing their loved ones. They showed grief and horror. I didn't know what to say to comfort them. I also knew that whatever I said couldn't pacify their soul. I felt for them.

Although I've practiced Buddhism, I felt powerless in this situation. There was so much suffering out there. How could I help? I didn't know.

Learn Your Suffering Patterns and
Stop Repeating Your Suffering

Many years ago, I started teaching meditation. I tried my best to help my students. No matter how hard I tried, no one understood what I said. I stopped the class after one year. Nevertheless, I still tried to communicate my knowledge to help my students whenever I had the chance. Although they all longed for happiness and freedom, and even though they really paid attention to what I said, even after 7 years they still couldn't understand me.

As a matter of fact, there is no method for meditation. Most people cannot understand meditation. They don't know how to do it. Many spiritual folks also don't know how to do it. I knew my students were working hard to practice what I said. However, they were still suffering. I felt heavy for this.

It is most difficult to understand your suffering patterns. Many people are suffering in their relationships. Take the relationship with your parents for example. You may have a good relationship with your parents for a while, and then it's not going so well for another time. Most people are suffering in these cycles. They cannot see their suffering patterns. Yet, once they spot their suffering patterns, these programs will stop eventually.

Images of all these people's suffering kept surfacing back to me when I was sitting quietly. However, I also knew that there was no effective meditation method that could free these people from their suffering. Because all these methods are designed by the mind, and the mind cannot free us from our mind.

Activating Your Inner Healing Power

One day, an inspiration came to me: Let's just release our own suffering patterns and follow them. Actually, to my own surprise, this method has proven very effective in releasing suffering. The Letting Go Method can activate your inner healing power and heal the suffering of your soul.

In the beginning, I just used it to release my own physical discomforts. I discovered that if I said the right releasing sentences, the discomfort started dissolving unless they were long term injuries. I then tried to release the emotional suffering patterns and to my own surprise, it works like magic! All you need to do is just to say the right releasing sentences.

At that time, I had spent a lot of time practicing Qigong and was very good at using it to heal physical discomfort for myself. However, I couldn't heal myself when physical discomfort was entangled with emotions and thoughts. Therefore, I applied this releasing method to all aspects of my life including body, relationships, and spirituality. I wanted to know how it can help us in different ways.

I worked tirelessly trying out this method on all aspects of my life no matter whether I was lying down, standing, or sitting. And then I discovered, it could work on complicated physical discomforts when they are related with emotions or thoughts. These are complicated suffering patterns.

After trying out The Letting Go Method for years, I have concluded that it is very effective in releasing our suffering. The Method can help us break through difficult suffering patterns. It can also help us discover our inner unconscious sufferings.

Releasing: Know Your True Feelings

It is impossible to heal your disease when the disease is entangled with your emotions. Body and emotions influence each other. The Method can heal both dimensions. It can also heal the stress and body discomfort like a frozen shoulder for example.

Learn from Your Relationships

The Method can not only help with body and emotional suffering, it can also help with entangled relationships. It's especially helpful for family relationships.

My son used to nag me a lot. He always told me what to do. It's almost like he was the senior and I was the junior. For example, he always complained that I did too many sitting sessions. He also often said to me, "How did you get you driver's license? You are such a terrible driver!" And I responded, "How dare you say that? You were not even born when I was driving around!"

I wasn't a Buddha yet. Sometimes his nagging made me upset. It was just that I recovered from my emotional outbreak very fast. One time, the same feeling surfaced again, so I decided to take a deep look at what was hiding over there. I watched this feeling. I was present with this feeling, and I released this feeling, and then the truth surfaced. The truth is that he loves me very much and that he would do everything, even sacrificing his life to keep me around. The truth is, he was crying and begging me not to leave!

At that special moment, I could sense his determination to keep me around. He was effectively saying, "As long as you stay around, I would do everything for you." I was very moved! He loves his mother. He wants to keep me around but he is not aware of how he really feels deep inside. Instead of expressing his love to me verbally, he nags me instead. What he is really looking for is to be loved and to be cared for!

I learned a lot from this insight. What can we learn from our relationship with our family? We need to understand our thinking patterns and not fall into the traps of our mind. Take my son's interaction with me for example. If I hadn't tried to understand the deep truth inside of him, we would have had a very tense relationship.

He is not into learning yet. If he were into learning, he would find out that the truth is, "I love my mom and I want to have my mom around." I always wanted to live in the mountains. I will drive deep to the mountains whenever I have a chance. No one knows where I am and there is no way to contact me. Sometimes he will say, "Will you be wolfed down by a bear?" What he really tries to express is that he really cares about me. Try to understand your thinking patterns. If my son could try to learn, understand his thinking patterns, and observe, he would find out that deep down he loves his mom very much. If he could know this truth, the way he would have interacted with me would have been different.

Be Thankful, Be Powerful

My elder sister passed away in 1993. She committed suicide. I was never willing to face this truth. She was ten years older than I am. I was almost brought up by her. She took care of me. She fed me and played with me. We had a very, very good relationship. I loved her very much and also depended on her very much.

I was not willing to face her death. I didn't even want to think about it, until one day I was willing to face the truth. I released this incident. My first reaction was anger, "How dare you leave me alone? How could you not love me anymore?" After the anger dissolved though, I felt calm. Still, it seemed like something was missing. I sat quietly with this feeling and let this feeling show me the way. Within less than a minute, gratitude surfaced deep from my soul!

What was I grateful for? I was grateful that she really cared for me. I was grateful that she loved me very deeply. I was grateful that there had been this wonderful person in my life! The gratitude kept bubbling up and dissolved all the anger, grief, and abandonment brought about by her death! And then I realized, she and I never separated. She is in my soul. She is in my heart. She is here with me forever! This lesson taught me the power of gratitude!

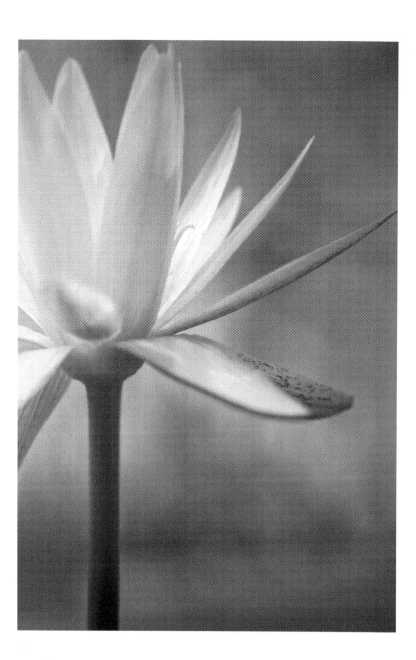

CHAPTER 3

The Letting Go Method

The Basic Principles of The Letting Go Method:

- Face your suffering patterns
- Be aware of your suffering patterns
- Let go of your suffering patterns

Why are we stuck in suffering? Why do we keep being stuck in a state of suffering at different times and in different situations?

The main reason that we resist our suffering is that we want to get rid of it. We often feel uneasy or are even scared when we feel anxious or restless. We mostly want to get rid of these feelings when they first arise. We go shopping, we gossip, we watch TV, we meditate, we chant, or we even recite mantras to get rid of this uneasiness. We may get temporary relief but the suffering is always there.

We are stuck in our suffering because we are running away from it.

Positive Affirmations

"Try to think positively." We hear that often. I am not saying that this is a bad method. However, it really clouds our consciousness.

My experience is that if we want to think positively when we feel sad, and say, "Don't feel sad. Let go! Letting go gives me the chance to grow and become powerful! Treat the experience as a present and be grateful for the people who hurt me," your grief will disappear for a moment, but it will come back at a later stage. Maybe it doesn't appear as sadness then but comes back as anger instead.

Positive thinking prevents us from digging deep into our consciousness and hence prevents us from finding the real cause of our sadness. Our real emotions hence bury themselves deep inside our soul. So, we need to understand that positive thinking is almost like running away from ourselves as well.

It is an okay method when you don't have enough energy to face your issues and transcend your suffering patterns. You need to have energy and strength to face your issues. What we are learning now is to accumulate the energy to face and deal with the real causes of our suffering.

Change Your Mindset: Negate and Repress Your Emotions

The so called "change your mindset" amounts effectively to repressing your emotions. For example, when you are angry you could tell yourself that you are a civilized person and you don't get angry. What you are really doing is thinking that you shouldn't get angry. The upset feelings don't disappear when you decide for them to do so.

We don't really know much about these negative emotions. As a matter of fact, anger or unease is just a different form of energy. It is a life force. It is a lively energy. When we repress our anger or unease all the time, eventually the sharpness, passion or liveliness will be gone as well. Eventually we will become stiff, slow, and then, sick.

As you can see here, changing our mindset or our attitude is not a good way to deal with our negative emotions. We can only transform our negative emotions by spending time with them, being with them, and understanding them. They can then be transformed to an energy of passion and liveliness. This is the procedure of The Letting Go Method.

Our emotions are our energy. If we cannot accept this energy, our strained faces will reflect the truth in a distorted way. If we cannot embrace everything in our life, and only accept positive, beautiful things, our heart becomes narrow and our life will be limited.

Put Down Your Thoughts: Get in Touch with Your True Self

Someone told me, "I can isolate my anger and not let it show in my life." As a matter of fact, she only thinks that she can live a life like that. The truth is that she leads a life far away from herself. She is always angry and talks to people with an angry voice. It is just that she has no idea what she is truly all about.

You cannot see your truth because there is a thinking process that is separate from the truth. You are very angry but you repress this truth. Eventually, you become detached from yourself and have no feelings left.

It is easy to look through your thoughts. Don't defend yourself and don't explain yourself. Don't be misled by your thoughts. You will get trapped whenever you try to analyze and think.

Changing your mindset is just like taking painkillers for your physical pain. You keep repressing your issues until you get really sick. What we need to do now is to look at ourselves. If there is a gap between us and our true self, it is caused by our thoughts.

Meditation: Let Your Suffering Pattern Be Present as It Is

People say, "If you can walk with peace and ease, where you are is heaven."

This is the same concept as changing your mindset. This is not learning about yourself. This is more like learning concepts and ideas.

"Walk with peace." How can you walk with peace when you have so many struggles inside? How do you feel when people tell you to feel peaceful when you are feeling turbulent instead? It's like you are very angry and people tell you to calm down. You can appear to be calm but inside of you a storm is brewing.

Meditation is to let your suffering pattern present itself as it is. When you let your suffering pattern present itself as it is, your suffering will disappear like a dark cloud releasing its dense structure with the rain and then dissolves. Maybe your dark cloud has ten layers. Just release them one by one. Then you will be able to see your suffering pattern present itself as it is. When you take this approach, your soul will gradually become clear. However, following the other popular concepts will not release your suffering patterns. It will only add an additional layer which weighs your soul down even more.

When you tell yourself that "I should…" and take action accordingly, you will feel better for maybe five minutes but soon you will feel just the same again. This is what a changed mindset does to you.

Meditation is taking the opposite route. You let your suffering present itself as it is. You experience your life storm as it is. Gradually, the storm disappears. All you need to do is pay attention and be alert when the storm presents itself.

Clear Your Suffering with Awareness: No More Accumulation of New Suffering

Recognizing the suffering and admitting it to yourself is the first step toward ending your suffering. Most people are scared to admit it to themselves. Most people think that if they admit something, it will put them in a bad situation like being inadequate, bad or vulnerable. Some other people associate admitting with owning the mess, punishment or repentance. Hence, they will resist and try to avoid admitting the suffering to themselves.

As a matter of fact, admitting it to yourself brings you the power to accept a situation from your heart. When you can truly admit something to yourself, your suffering can come to an end. Then it is possible to have a new beginning. That being said, only when you are able to admit it to yourself, can you put your suffering patterns to an end. Otherwise, these sufferings will always follow you.

When you admit something to yourself, you start the process of clearing up the pain. Take guilt for example. Once you admit guilt's existence, all the related entanglements will present themselves because when you admit it, you clear up a space for things to happen. You need to do all these things with awareness, or you have to keep clearing up these sufferings because you keep creating new ones.

The first step of clearing up your sufferings starts with stopping to accumulate new causes. To achieve this goal, we need to be aware all the time. Whatever method we take to liberate ourselves from suffering; the common method is the awareness of all our inner workings. If we don't clear up our sufferings with the help of awareness, all our healing attempts will be meaningless.

It is very difficult to stay aware because we easily fall victim to our thinking patterns. We take everything that happens within us for granted. I want to remind you all here, please, don't take anything for granted. Once you take all these inner workings for granted, you become dull.

Letting Go: Inquire About the Truth Beneath the Appearance

With the help of The Letting Go Method we are able to see our suffering patterns. The reason to release these suffering patterns is not to make them vanish yet but first to understand them. When we can see the truth beneath our suffering, true love will arise in our relationships. We will then stop manipulating each other in the name of love.

Love is not "I love you and you love me." Love is that we learn to connect and communicate with each other through these suffering patterns. If you don't try to understand your suffering, you will always feel lonely in your relationships. You don't feel love in your relationships because these suffering patterns prevent you from experiencing it. In this situation, you will only feel frustrated if you keep demanding love from others or work so hard to please them.

My son used to spend a lot of time playing video games. The time he spent on the internet was getting longer and longer. I tried all kinds of methods to keep him from the electronic devices. Actually, the motivation behind my behavior was fear. I worried that his eyes would get bad. I worried that it would hinder his academic success. So, what I was effectively doing by nagging was making sure these things wouldn't happen, so that I could reassure myself.

So first came the worry, then came the reassurance to make myself feel secure. What I was effectively doing was keeping myself from worrying. It was primarily out of my own needs and only secondarily out of my child's needs.

Whenever we want our children or partner to do something to make us feel secure, we are often motivated by our old injuries. Once we can see that we are doing things as a result of our old injuries, we can use The Letting Go Method to release them. Only when we can release ourselves from what is holding us back can we have real freedom.

The Letting Go Order: External to Internal

Imagine that you throw a pebble into a peaceful lake. Immediately, the lake is full of ripples. This is how The

Letting Go Method functions. We confront our soul with issues just like throwing a pebble into a peaceful lake. How big the pebble is and how deep the pebble can go will decide how widespread and how big the ripples will be.

It's very important to stay present when the lake is full of ripples because your obstacles won't exist by themselves. The problem you are currently facing is connected with all other problems. Stay present when you are practicing The Letting Go Method.

What Are Letting Go Sentences?

All words that we speak out loud manifest as energy. All energy is a magnetic field. Letting Go Sentences are not mantras. There is deep meaning associated with these sentences. All the sound waves can penetrate our energy field. When we speak out the Letting Go Sentences, we are using sound energy to invoke the flowing of our energy field.

Our sound is a wave—an energy—and so is our pain. Whenever you speak out these Letting Go Sentences, you are using the sound wave to initiate another wave movement.

You can start with an easy emotion. For example, if you feel bored and don't know the reason, you can try to let go of the energy of being bored. You can also pay attention to things that you are interested in doing or having. For example, if you have an eating disorder, you can try to let go of the energy of overeating or eating too little. This will be the beginning sentence for the Letting Go Method. And then you pay attention to your feelings and thoughts that pop to the surface after practicing the first Letting Go Sentence. You can also let go of the energy of foot ache, knee pain, back ache, or a headache. The key is to observe and pay attention to our problems.

The Steps of The Letting Go Method

There are no fixed steps for The Letting Go Method. All you need to do is speak out the emotions or issues that you want to let go of. For example, "Let go of the energy of losing my loved one." It will then open a door for you.

In the beginning, we usually let go of our thoughts. Slowly, we learn to let go of our emotions and then we let go of the root cause of our suffering. Whenever you speak out the right Letting Go Sentences, you can always feel the feedback from your body. You will experience a lot of emotions when you are practicing The Letting Go Method. For example, if your Letting Go Sentence is, "Don't leave me alone", you will feel abandoned and left behind. Even it's just a short sentence, the intensive pain you experience is just like someone punching you right on the chest.

Question: "My chest feels really painful whenever I am practicing The Letting Go Method and no matter how I try to let go, my chest still really hurts. What should I do?"

This is because the energy associated with your obstacle will be stuck in the weaker spots of your body, like your heart for example. All the stuck energy is stored there. You cannot heal this kind of ache by just seeing a doctor. You have to take care of this ache by seeing a doctor and healing your emotional pain as well. If you can find the corresponding Letting Go Sentence, the stuck energy in this spot will start to loosen up. As a matter of fact, if we can be very relaxed and open, whenever we are practicing The Letting Go Method, the energy will lead us to the corresponding sentences. We empathize with our own pain during the process of letting go.

Starting from the External Obstacles

All emotions are energy waves. These energy waves are like the rainbow. When you practice The Letting Go Method, you have to start letting go of the obstacles ranging from external to internal causes. Don't rush to the root cause in the beginning. This is just like dressing in layers of clothes when we go out into the freezing weather. Now we are going inside the house—should we take off the inside layer first or the outside layer first?

Someone may feel cold again after undressing just one layer. Someone else has to stop after taking off two layers. Another person can keep undressing himself beyond three layers. He will only stop undressing when he feels the temperature is just right.

When you are letting go of your obstacles, attention and stillness are key. Adopt the attitude of "knowing your obstacles" instead of "how it should be", i.e., allow every condition and message as you receive it. There is no other intention in your practice other than to know yourself. In this way, your obstacles will be reduced layer by layer by themselves.

In a word, all you need to do is to just pay attention without doing anything. You may have a big reaction when you let go of big issues like fear or emptiness. This is because you came across these issues in all of your past lives. After you let go of these fears and this emptiness, your life is no longer driven by them and you can finally live your life and learn!

Connecting with Yourself Is Key

Stay open while you are releasing your suffering. Don't set up any specific intentions. Just stay naturally alert and present. With this natural alertness, you will discover and recognize your thought patterns at work, as well as witness the emotions related to your suffering.

These thoughts show up while you are releasing your suffering. You have concluded this after experiencing different life events and you have been living your life according to these conclusions. For example, sometimes you feel powerless. You are not stuck in the feeling of being powerless. It's just a thought. To the contrary, you have been feeling this way because you have been experiencing a lot and your mind has been trying to intervene in your life for way too long.

You have been feeling powerless because you have been making a lot of efforts. You have been thinking a lot about your life. You have been experiencing many emotions, and you have had many different experiences. All of these together create the feeling of being powerless. We cannot just get rid of this feeling. We can only pay attention to it gradually. If we cannot understand what causes this feeling of powerlessness, it will resurface again and again.

Your attention to yourself is your doorway to connect with yourself. Almost all of us have created an image of ourselves and we lead our lives accordingly. We think that living up to this image will mean that we are accepted and appreciated, that we will be loved and get recognition. The motivation behind this thought is fear. If you don't connect with yourself, you won't be able to discover how your suffering patterns function. Hence, you cannot see your own truth. In this way, you will feel alienated. You won't understand why you are doing these things and why you are saying these words.

Meditation teaches us how to express ourselves as is. Once you can see how your mind tricks you, you don't need to wear these masks and fall for these images.

Release Your Old Wounds

If you have some old injuries, get back to the original incident. Release the original image and release that old wound. You can apply the same techniques to your emotional injuries.

For example, when you feel grief, release the energy of grief. Once you start releasing this grief energy, the energy will be activated and becomes fluid. Consequently, relevant incidents and images will start showing up. You can temporarily stay in this state for a while. This will probably last for one or two minutes and then the grief energy will start to flow.

There will be many thoughts that show up while this energy is flowing. Pay attention to them. Be mindful to what kind of thoughts arise. Also, be aware how you react to these thoughts. These thoughts are running your life. Maybe they don't show up directly as grief. They could show up as your way of responding to challenges in life. Be aware and stay alert.

How It comes, How It Goes

When you are releasing your suffering, you may start to cough, yawn, or lose your focus. This is because the negative energies are releasing, or are trying to find a new place to stay.

Your whole energy field is circulating all the time. Whenever any emotion gets stuck in you, the energy stays in the weakest part of your system. That's why someone starts coughing when they get angry. Other people get diarrhea when they get upset. If you yawn, it means that you don't have enough oxygen in your brain. When the negative energy stays in your brain, you will have trouble sleeping. Either your sleep quality is poor, or you have difficulty falling asleep. You could also feel like you never get enough sleep. If you cough, it means that this negative energy stays in your respiratory system or lungs.

How it comes, so it goes. This negative energy doesn't get stuck in our system without reason. When we are releasing our suffering, as we get better physically and emotionally, the same negative energy will be released from our system.

Who Is Experiencing Suffering? Who Is Feeling Sad?

Don't think about getting rid of your suffering. By practicing The Letting Go Method, your suffering will dissolve by itself. The exercise is much more efficient than thinking about how to get rid of it. All you need to do is release these different kinds of energy, and stay aware. Observation will arise by itself when you are doing this exercise.

The Four Stages of The Letting Go Method

First, when we practice The Letting Go Method, negative energy will start to be released and you may feel like crying or like having been wronged. All you need to do at this stage is just stay relaxed.

33

Second, the content of this suffering or the injury will start to show up. Just stay relaxed and do nothing. Follow the emerging feeling.

Third, the thought patterns, mind creations, or undertaken efforts will start to show up. Just stay present and let them show up by themselves. Either a physical or mental negative energy will surface. Just allow it.

Fourth, inquire about your suffering. For example, I often ask my students, "Who is accusing?" Just stay present and don't use your mind. The person who is feeling sad may surface in response to the question. If you use your mind, you just couldn't figure out how these two can be linked together. But the truth is, accusing and sadness are just like two sides of a coin.

Stay present with all your inquiries without the intervention of your mind. It's very powerful when you stay present. All the deep buried suffering may show up when you are present. At this moment, when you ask yourself "Who is feeling sad?", you may see from your internal image that you lost someone or learn something about an occurrence in one of your past lives. You may totally break down at this moment. After your breakdown, you will feel alive again! Let the hurt of that past life flow! Let the loss and suffering of that past life be seen! Only after that are you able to live again!

Alternate Between The Letting Go Method and Inquiry

Say you feel abandoned or despised, all of these emotions arise from prior injuries, but most of the time you don't know what these injuries are. After you release the energy of feeling despised three or four times ask yourself, "Who is feeling despised?" This question will act like dropping a rock into a quiet lake. Just wait to see what kind of ripples will surface.

Maybe you feel despised because you didn't have good grades when you were little. Maybe your family was poor when you were young. You may have felt ashamed when people despised you. You can then release the energy of feeling shameful. This shameful energy is an injury. It stays in your consciousness. How much you can bear of this shameful energy decides how well you can heal yourself.

You can use The Letting Go Method with people, events or things. When you inquire, "Who is feeling despised?", an alien version of yourself may show up. This person may be different than how you feel like you are at this moment. Whatever shows up, just release it. Your suffering will dissolve by itself.

Inquire, release; release, inquire. This method is very simple. The difficult part is if we don't have awareness and stillness, we cannot catch and follow the whole process until the end. We may stop the process in the middle.

Be Present Without the Motivation
to Get Rid of Your Suffering

When we feel pain, our first reaction is to get rid of it. When you have a stomach ache, you go and see a doctor. You take medicine and you want to get rid of your pain. The same applies to mental suffering. We just want to get rid of it as soon as possible.

You will walk on the wrong path when your motivation is to get rid of your pain. It's like you want to get rid of your fear of insecurity so you work hard to succeed. The motivation to get rid of fear creates a lot of desires in us.

When you are not afraid of being small, you won't need to prove yourself. When you don't have any opinion about gain or loss, you don't need to work desperately to succeed. When you want to succeed, the fear of failure arises too. When you want to be respected, the fear of being small will also arise. When you want to get rid of suffering, your life keeps being entangled with suffering.

The motivation to get rid of suffering is the movement of the mind. It is driven by will. It is a promise to yourself created by your mind. Only when you stop the motivation, you can feel the stillness and stability. When the stillness arises, you can liberate yourself from the limitation of yourself and get to a place where the mind cannot touch you.

Take letting go of the energy of self-pity as an example. When we start to release the energy of self-pity, there will be several different wavelengths and energies that come to the surface. These energies will start flowing. However, if the motivation to get rid of suffering is too strong, since the motivation is a mind movement, this motivation will influence the releasing waves as well. The wave will become weak and cannot release much suffering energy.

The primary function of being present with your suffering is not to get rid of your suffering, but instead to discover the insight, "My mind creates this suffering; it is not real." For example, I was very sick before and my mind created a belief set that I needed to do my best to prevent myself from getting sick again. As a result, this belief set created more belief sets and actions. Hence, I was suffering even more because of this belief set.

You are not present with your suffering because you want to get rid of your suffering. To truly be present with your suffering means that you know that this suffering is an illusion and that you are not against this suffering. Nor do you try to diminish it.

Stop and Be Present with Intensive Attention

After you speak out one Letting Go Sentence, stop and be present. What thought surfaces? What response do you have? To stop and be present is the key for practicing The Letting Go Method.

For example, after we release the energy of self-blaming, stop and pay attention to what kind of energy shows up. It may be frustrated energy or angry energy. We don't know what kind of energy will show up. We also don't know when it will show up. When it surfaces, you will feel uncomfortable, exhausted, or experience different kinds of pain.

The pain may stay for three seconds, four seconds, or five seconds. And then another strong emotion may surface. It may be the energy of wanting to be recognized, the desire to succeed or the feeling of guilt. Stay and be present with this state for a while. Let the energy finish its own cycle. Don't deliberately look for these energies. Let them flow naturally instead. When the course is finished, you will feel relaxed. Suddenly, you realize that your obstacle is gone or has become weak. We can recognize it next time when it shows up, not by our mind but by its energy.

While you pay full attention and are present while practicing The Letting Go Method, your mind stops. At that moment, your suffering and your issues start to change. Also, you see through your reality. This is the essence of practicing this method.

When we face our sufferings, even when we think that they are ugly and imperfect, it may not be the truth. These sufferings are only ugly and imperfect in our mind's opinion. It may not be the truth. After you speak out the Letting Go Sentence, how are you at that moment? Your full attention with your issues can dissolve them. You can only know your truth at this moment, and not your mind.

We feel pain because we relive the past in the present moment. Our memory and response still stay in the moment when we were wounded. We remember them and use the same interpretation to respond in the present moment. We have no idea that we are influenced by our past and project it to the future. In this way, our obstacles and fears are taking deep root in us.

When we are letting go of the past obstacles, the point is not to relive the past but to recognize that this moment is different from the moment you were wounded but you are still influenced by the past moment. When you see that, your suffering starts dissolving. The point is not about what to do, or practice a certain way, but to pay attention to your response. How do you respond to the incidents in your life? How do you respond to your thoughts? How do you respond to the things and the people around you?

If you cannot stay present, you will relive your patterns. Your patterns are not new. They are always from experiences and concepts from the past. Your responses from the dead experiences or concepts are the shadows of the past and cannot be new or creative. Our life and relationships are happening in the present moment. When we respond to them with our past experiences, we cannot recognize the truth of this present moment or the present issue. This is the main reason that we cannot communicate with each other in our relationships.

Love Is to Know Your Suffering Patterns

"He shouldn't treat me like this. If he hadn't treated me like this, I wouldn't behave like this." What's this? This is concept and thought! If you keep letting your mind control your relationship, the suffering will stay with you for a while.

To heal your pain and suffering, love is the only medicine. If you truly loved a person, you wouldn't put up conditions such as loving them only if your demands are satisfied Can we apply the same attitude to our suffering and pain? How do you feel when you love your suffering and pain?

When you don't feel well, just follow the feeling. Be present with the feeling. Don't think, "He shouldn't have treated me like this." Neither will accepting the pain come to your mind. You will just allow yourself to be miserable, totally miserable. No thoughts. Neither accept it or reject it. Just be with it.

No more feelings of hatred, guilt, or smallness towards our suffering. No more demanding or fighting against our suffering. Love arises in us when we know ourselves. Love isn't just a noun. We are love.

Be Present with Your Movement: Be Present with Your Suffering

We need a lot of energy to face our bigger issues and our deep suffering patterns. If you are not learning, you cannot pay attention. You cannot look deeply and you cannot see broadly. You have a lot of struggles and many concepts, and the struggles between your concepts and your ideas will drain your energy. Hence, you don't have the energy to face your real issues and can only stay in a state of suffering, sadness, anger, hatred and violence.

By being aware of your daily movement, like the movement of your hands or feet, you can accumulate your energy. Awareness feeds stillness. When stillness arises in you regularly, you will naturally have the ability to face your issues and suffering patterns.

Walking Meditation

When you walk, before you put down your feet, use the middle inner side of your foot as a baseline. First, let your sole touch the ground, and then the middle part, and then your toes. Place your feet on the ground using this pattern.

Every time you put down your foot, know that you are putting down your foot on the ground. Every time you raise your foot, know that you are raising your foot. So, you are aware that you are raising your foot from the ground, or putting down your foot on the ground.

Raise your head and look straight. Be aware whenever you raise your foot. Be aware whenever you put down your foot. Now pay attention to your shoulder. Relax your shoulder. Stay present with your foot activity of putting it down and raising it up again.

Relax your shoulders. Let go of all the issues. Be present with every step of raising your foot and be present with your every step of putting down your foot. Relax your shoulders.

Now listen to the sounds around you. Listen to the wind. Be aware of your foot's movement; one, two, three. Listen to the sounds around you. Be aware that you are raising up your foot; one, two, three. Relax your shoulders. One, two, three; you raise your foot; one, two, three, you put down your foot. Listen to the sounds around you.

Relax your shoulders. Listen to the sounds around you. Listen to the wind. Listen to the tree leaves swaying. One, two, three; know that you are putting down your foot; one, two, three; know that you are raising your foot. Listen to the sounds around you. Relax your shoulders. How are you walking? Are you feeling stiff?

Relax your shoulders

Be aware of your body. Is there any area where you feel tense? In the meantime, be aware that you are raising your foot and putting it down afterwards. Listen to the sounds around you. Listen to your inner voice. Listen to your inner voice just like you are listening to the wind, just like you are aware that you are lifting up your foot and putting it down. Listen!

Relax your shoulders. Listen to your inner voice. Listen to the wind. Listen to the swaying leaves. Listen to your inner voice. Be aware of the movement of raising up and putting down your foot. Be aware of every movement of raising up and putting down your foot. Let this awareness act just like you are listening. Listen to your foot being raised up. Listen to your foot being put down.

Raise your head. Raise your chest. Relax your shoulders. Listen to the sounds around you. Listen to the sound of raising your body parts. Listen. Listen to your inner voice.

Relax your shoulders. Okay, stop right there. Feel your body. Feel your shoulders. Move your shoulders a little bit. How did you feel when you were walking just now? What thoughts came to your mind?

Be aware if you try to intervene with your thoughts. Pay attention to the thoughts arising in you just like when you are paying attention to your movements of raising up and putting down your foot. Be with yourself silently. Be with your thoughts as they arise quietly. Be with the feelings as they arise in you silently just like when you are listening to the wind. Just listen. Just like when you are aware of your movement of raising up and putting down your foot. Just be aware.

Listen Without Your Mind

What is listening?

We never really listen to each other. When we really listen, time stills. What does this really mean? Say, when we are listening to the rain and the rain drops are falling. We don't have any expectation of how the rain drops should fall. We have no preference about the rain. At this moment, only the rain is present. The person who is listening to the rain disappears. In this situation, time stills.

When we can listen like this, we become sharp, clear and enlightened. However, once the "I"—thought and should—appears, it becomes crowded and busy. When we just listen without the "I", the ability to be aware arises.

When you can be aware with clarity, you will be aware immediately when the "I" shows up. This immediate awareness brings out your insights. You don't have your insights by reading a book. You don't get your insights from school but from pure listening. When pure listening arises within you, you have the chance to liberate yourself from your "I". You become liberated from your mind, liberated from the challenges of life. You can only know your conditioning and mind in this pure state.

Just listen. Listen to any sound. Be aware of how you listen. What kind of feelings arise in you? What thoughts arise in you? Just be aware without taking any action. It's really important to be aware of the rising thoughts. Every thought is connected to another. With this attention, a different energy field is created, and insights arise free from the "I".

How are you when you are listening? Are your anger or grief sufferings still there? When you are listening, they stop temporarily. They are not functioning at that moment. You are not listening with your anger. You are not listening with your grief. You are not using your mind to listen.

Listening without our mind opens up our self-sufficient energy. The heart is still. The senses get even sharper and clearer. No intervention. It is a pure and unknown state. At this moment, we enter another space, another dimension. We are connected with energy from another dimension. The energy cleansing happens by itself at this moment. The cleansing process is intensified if you speak the Letting Go Sentences.

No Escape: No Indulgence

Once your attention is off, your releasing movement is interrupted as well. Why is your attention off? Because you feel that you have had enough and that you cannot deal with it anymore. Perhaps there is something in life you cannot handle anymore. You will find that you have a similar reaction when you practice meditation. You feel restless. "I don't want to sit here anymore. I want to stop now." Every time you come across obstacles, you want to run away.

Many factors decide your ability to sit still. It's not just an expression of willpower. The deeper your stillness is, the deeper you are able to deal with your obstacles. You have to upgrade your ability in different aspects to deal with different obstacles.

"I thought the reason I wanted to stop my sitting meditation is because I already sat for 30-60 minutes. I don't think I wanted to stand up because I wanted to stop meditation but because my mind started getting restless. Also, my back got sore".

We always think that this is the reason that forces us to stop our sitting meditation, but the truth is that it is not. The same applies to our response to issues that arise in our relationships. We just break up, leave, or get angry. The reason is that our attention is off while we are practicing releasing. It is just like the energy is getting obstructed while flowing. Your response to obstacles in your life is the same. You cannot keep going while sitting. You cannot keep going while practicing The Letting Go Method. The same applies if you cannot stay in your relationship when you come across difficulties. This is your pattern to obstacles in your life. If we cannot see through this pattern and let go of this pattern, this pattern will stay with us.

You can only change your fate by staying aware in your life.

Enjoy the Clouds

When we look at the clouds, why are we in awe of their beauty? Why don't we appreciate our own beauty when we are looking at ourselves?

"I can control myself but I cannot control the clouds."

Can you control yourself? Can you decide what thoughts arise in you? Can you decide how you will respond to certain situations? Can you control your mind and suffering? Why do we have so much "should, identification, and thought" when we are looking at ourselves?

We are objective when we are looking at the clouds. We are subjective when we are looking at ourselves.

That's right. When we are looking at the clouds, we just appreciate them. No matter how they change, they are still beautiful! When we are looking at ourselves, our mind starts intervening, "No, I have to be like this or that." Can we apply the same attitude when we look at our suffering? In this way, our suffering will be as beautiful as the clouds.

You can have the same attitude, not only while enjoying the clouds. You can have this attitude even with walking, or with work. The problem is not with the clouds. The problem is not with the change. The problem is with our attitude—not to interfere, not to control. Let's be open to ourselves just like we are open to the clouds. Then we will be as beautiful as the clouds are every day.

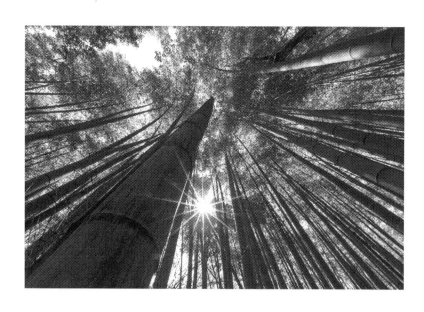

CHAPTER 4

Practice The Letting Go Method

CHAPTER 4.1

Get Ready

1. Create a comfortable and quiet space. Give yourself 50 minutes of free time

2. You can read out these Letting Go Sentences, prerecord these sentences, or have someone who can focus and sympathize read them for you. Pause 10 seconds to 30 seconds between each sentence. Pause, relax, and pay attention to your body and emotional responses after you read out each sentence. Keep your awareness passive. Allow your emotions to flow and release. Allow yourself to cry.

3. The energy flow of the different Letting Go Sentences will be different for each person. If you have a strong reaction to a certain sentence, stay there for a while. Be aware of the thoughts and the images that emerge. If some strong and vivid emotional experiences show up, just release these

emotions and experiences first. You don't need to finish all the Letting Go Sentences. You can release whatever emotions surface up. Release them layer by layer.

4. It's natural to get distracted by particular issues or memories. Just bring yourself back to the release exercise after you notice that you are distracted.

5. People who are used to repressing their anger may feel like shouting. Just allow yourself to shout; stomp your feet, punch the pillows. If you can always express your unhappiness, feel yourself quietly when you read out these sentences and allow the pain beneath the anger to surface.

6. You may feel like hiccupping or yawning. You may experience a stomach ache or feel blank after the energy starts to flow. There is no need to worry too much about these reactions.

7. Prepare paper and pen and write down your discovery while practicing your releasing exercises. Remember, the quality of your attention is much more important than the content that you have discovered.

Drop Your Effort—Daily Life Letting Go Practices

Connect with Your Body

Past memories will show up when you are meditating with a relaxed body and your mind is quiet. This is very beautiful. These memories surface to help us heal. Face them and stop your resistance.

We all have been hurt. These injuries may take the form of verbal abuse, or feeling lost, fear or grief, and so forth. If we never face them, they will accumulate and store in our body. Over time this will make us sick or sore. Right now, at this moment, I invite you to connect with your body.

Let us start noticing our body's existence.

Please say to your body, "Sorry that I ignored you."

Let your mouth face toward your chest and say, "Sorry, sorry, sorry! I will be with you from now on."

Relax your shoulders and say, "Sorry, sorry. I will be with you from now on."

Relax your shoulders and say, "Sorry. I will be with you from now on."

Relax your shoulders and release your efforts.

Now, slowly apologize to the areas that often feel unwell. Maybe it is your waist, or your back. Say, "Sorry, sorry, that I ignored you."

"Sorry, sorry, that I ignored you. I will be with you from here on. I will be with you from now on."

With love, say, "I am with you now."

With love, say, "I am with you now."

Relax your shoulders, move your mouth toward your chest, and with love say, "I am with you now."

Now imagine these areas that are often unwell. Imagine that there is a ray of very gentle, very bright golden light right above your head. It surrounds your body and slowly flows through all the unwell areas. This healing energy flows to wherever it is needed.

Do it one more time. Imagine that there is a ray of very gentle, very bright golden light right above your head, surrounding your body, slowly flowing through the unwell areas. It flows to wherever the healing energy is needed.

Say to your body, "Thank you!"

With your mouth moving towards your chest, say to your body, "Thank you! Thank you!"

The Listening Practice

Sit relaxed. Pay attention to your shoulders. Pay attention to your body. Sit straight without effort. Relax. Sit relaxed. Sit quietly.

Pay attention to your feet. Are they tight? Relax them. Release the tension. Pay attention to your calves. Release the tension. Pay attention to your knees. Pay attention to your thighs, release the tension. Pay attention to your pelvis.

Once again, relax your feet. Relax your legs. Release the tension. Say thank you to your feet and legs. Be with them. Listen to them. Tell them, "Thank you for taking me this far! Thank you for taking me to all the places I've dreamed of." Be with them!

Relax your shoulders. Relax your shoulders. Pay attention to your arms. Release your strength. Be with your shoulders. Express your gratitude to them.

Sit quietly. Listen to what surfaces within. What thoughts arise? Check if your body is tight. Relax your body. Relax the tension. Listen to what arises in you. Listen to your body!

"Should" does not exist. There is no "yes" or "no" either. Just listen. Listen to the voice coming from your mind. Listen to the reaction from your mind. There is no "how". Just listen.

Listen to your thoughts. Listen to each one of them. Listen to your reactions. These reactions are the root cause of our suffering.

Listen to the voice coming from your mind. Our suffering comes from this voice. Listen to this voice without choosing anything. Listen to these inner voices passively. Listen to these inner voices without having any intention. Listen to your voice without any effort. Listen to them silently.

Listen to anything the voice comes up with. Listen to the sound when the voice stops. Listen to the sound when the voice stops.

Know Your Effort

To make a living we of course need to work quite hard. However, many people work to get recognition, find acceptance, or to be superior. They always demand of themselves to do more and to do better. When you are on a cycle like this, your work is not just work. Your work is there to fill a hole inside. Effort like this only creates stress and frustration.

When your effort to work hard originates from the feeling of lack, or to seek recognition, whether you reach your ideal position or not, you will always be stressed and feel frustrated. At this moment, your effort becomes an obstacle to success. Once you have this realization, your work becomes effortless. You work efficiently, and you can reach your potential. Your performance is even better than you expect. At this moment, whatever you do is not reflecting your pain. Instead, you work because you are willing to work. You work because you want to work and you like to work. Since you are doing things you enjoy, you won't have the pressure to achieve something or get something.

So, what we focus on here is the mental effort. There is no doubt that you should work hard to make a living. What becomes bothersome though is the mental effort and the entanglement in interpersonal relationships.

Work to Get Recognition

When you are young, you study hard to impress your teachers and parents. After you grow up, you work hard to impress your friends, co-workers, supervisor, or your significant other. We work hard to fit in. We work hard to please. Why do we work so hard? How do you feel when you are accepted and recognized? You are loved. When you get an A+, your dad praises you. You then feel loved and secure. So, you work even harder to meet your parents' expectations.

We are subconsciously driven by the feeling of mental lack to seek love and security. We are scared of feeling empty. To fill this emptiness, we bury ourselves in work or get addicted to social media. If you can try to get to the root of this empty feeling, to know yourself as you truly are, and can finally get along with yourself, you can liberate yourself from this effort.

Many spiritual folks come across emptiness but most of them only know emptiness as a mind concept. "I know it. I know that there is emptiness inside me." Then there are some folks willing to face their emptiness but they are not able to transcend it. Therefore, when we practice letting go of emptiness, please hang out with this emptiness for a while. Let your body and soul merge with this emptiness and fear. Soon we will be able to get out of this prison.

Practicing The Letting Go Method liberates us from our thinking, and liberates us from our mind. It is a very interesting experience. Please experience it yourself. Maybe your mind cannot understand what I am saying but your heart will understand.

Effort Out of Guilt

Some effort is out of guilt. You work hard and sacrifice yourself to atone for your sins. You may even not remember what causes you to make this effort. However deep down in our subconsciousness resides guilt. We carry this energy with us to seek balance in our relationships. When we work to atone, we feel safe and painful at the same time. We are full of conflicts and struggles.

"I don't want to be like this", we say, or "I don't know what to do with him." Many people are stuck in this kind of relationship pattern. Even though they feel tired, they still work hard to atone themselves. There is no end for this suffering. People stuck in this pattern don't know how to liberate themselves from it. When we try to understand guilt and redemption, what will surface? Fear! Maybe this guilt is from our past lives. Maybe it's from our childhood. Maybe you carry the energy of guilt from your family. Whoever or wherever it is from, if it's in you, you need to work on it. Sometimes, it just happens. Just learn to let go of this energy.

Effort to Improve Self Confidence

Many people work hard because they feel that they are not good enough. They feel that they are not as good as others. They force themselves and demand of themselves to get better. In the end, they always feel powerless and frustrated. During the process to improve ourselves, we hurt ourselves mentally and physically. We have to release these injuries. We have to let go of the frustrated feelings that have accumulated over time. The energy of frustration drives negative mental and emotional energy to our physical body and makes us sick.

Why are we willing to suffer? We suffer because we want to be loved. We suffer because we want to feel secure. We suffer because we want to be needed. We suffer because we want to raise our self-confidence. However, do we really know what love, security and self-confidence is? Do we really know these states? Are we aware of what exactly we making an effort for?

There is stress accompanied with every effort. Even though you get something for your hard work, soon you will feel exhausted. Life is not a 100-meter sprint. Life is a marathon. You have to adjust your speed so you can stay on this journey longer. Too much effort makes people frustrated. Once you feel frustrated, your emptiness and fear will deepen because you don't have any extra energy to deal with it.

Because of your inner emptiness and fear, you need love and security. You don't have the need to work hard once your emptiness and fear disappears. After that, everything comes naturally to you.

Effort to Help People

Some people work hard to help people. This effort originates from their injuries and limitations. They can only feel fulfilled and powerful when they are helping others. There is a problem here. If you can only be happy by helping other people, why aren't you happy yourself?

Why do you feel happy when others express their gratitude? Why do you feel upset if they don't give you any positive feedback? Isn't it our own business whether we are happy or not?

We can see our own issues when we are practicing The Letting Go Method. How deep your healing can go depends on your ability to stay still. You are able to see, to accept, and to feel when you are able to stay still. As your energy starts to flow, soon you will realize that you look like you are helping others when actually you are just doing this for yourself. When you can see through all these issues originating from yourself, the energy you have toward others can be released.

Effort for Enlightenment

Some people work hard to become enlightened. They practice tirelessly to advance. However, do you think that you can get enlightenment by working hard? Obviously not. As a matter of fact, effort for enlightenment is the same as working hard to help people or to improve your self-confidence. You want to get enlightenment to get recognition, respect and power. How do you feel after you experience these feelings? Pleasure. Why do you need to feel pleasure? Because you feel empty.

We don't know how to deal with our empty feeling so we work in the opposite direction. If we can face this difficulty, our life will be different. We can also have a good influence on the people around us when we are at peace with ourselves. Why do we repeat our suffering? We repeat our suffering because we don't know any better. We repeat our suffering because of ignorance.

We don't know ourselves. We don't know our mind. When we have no idea what we are doing, even if we have already repeated our suffering a million times, we will still repeat it. Knowing yourself empowers you with the ability to liberate yourself from suffering and hence brings out the good influence you can have on the people around you.

Practice Letting Go of Your Effort

The most important thing in practicing The Letting Go Method is to stay still. Try to be aware of your mind and the thoughts that arise in you. Pay attention to your movements. However, when you cannot remain in this state and your thoughts arise, just be aware. There is no need to bring back the thoughts to your attention after they pass.

Listen to the sounds around you. Relax your shoulders.

Let go of the energy to make an effort. Relax your shoulders.

Let go of the person who is making the effort.

Let go of the person who is making the effort.

Let go of the hardworking person.

Let go of the person who works tirelessly.

Let go of the hardworking person.

Let go of the person who is swallowing all the humiliation.

Let go of the person who is swallowing all the humiliation.

Relax your shoulders.

Let go of the person who is unjustly treated.

Let go of the person who is unfairly treated.

Let go of the energy of being disapproved of.

Relax the shoulders.

Let go of the energy of having a heartache.

Let go of the energy of being heartbroken.

Let go of the energy of having a heartache.

Let go of the energy of being heartbroken.

Let go of the person with the heartache.

Let go of the person with the heartache.

Let go of the person with the heartache.

Let go of the frustrated person.

Let go of the frustrated person.

Let go of the frustrated person.

Let go of the frustrated person.

Let go of the frustrated person.

Let go of the energy of feeling frustrated.

Let go of the energy of feeling lost.

Let go of the lost person.

Relax your shoulders.

Let go of the lost person.

Let go of the lost person.

Who is lost?

Who is lost?

Relax your shoulders.

Let go of the person who lost everything.

Let go of the person who has nothing.

Let go of the empty energy.

Let go of the empty energy.

Be aware of the thoughts as they arise.

Let go of the empty energy.

Be aware of the appearing thoughts.

Let go of the empty energy.

Be with this energy.

Be with the emptiness.

Let go of the empty energy.

Let go of the empty energy.

Be aware of your appearing thoughts.

Let go of your empty energy.

Let go of the person who feels empty.

Let go of the negative energy in your right atrium.

Let go of the negative energy in your left atrium.

Be aware of your appearing thoughts.

Who is feeling lost?

Let go of the headache energy.

Let go of the person who is feeling empty.

Who is feeling empty?

Be aware of your appearing thoughts.

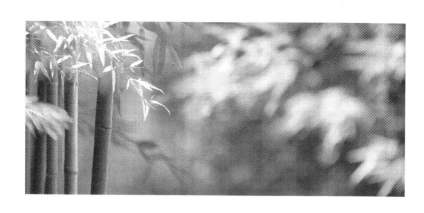

CHAPTER 4.2

Let Go of the Empty Energy

When you ask the question, "Who is feeling empty?", you need only to wait patiently for the answers. The energy will start flowing and show you the answers. Some past events, old injuries, or forgotten energy will surface. Please don't use your mind to get the answers. Please don't guess the answers. All you need to do is just ask the questions. The energy will surface by itself.

When our heart is open, all the energy that is buried deep down subconsciously will gradually surface. It will start flowing. If we want to understand it and be with it, it will heal itself.

Whenever you ask the question "who?", all you need to do is to wait quietly. Please don't have any assumption of what it will be. It may be something we forgot, something we cannot come up with or something that happened before that will surface. All we need to do is just wait quietly.

Let go of the empty energy.

Let go of the person who is feeling empty.

Who is feeling empty?

Who is feeling empty and lost?

Let go of the person who is left behind.

Let go of the energy of being left behind.

Be aware of the arising thoughts.

Let go of the empty energy.

Let go of the person who is feeling empty.

Be aware of the arising thoughts.

Let go of the empty energy.

Who is feeling empty?

For inquiry, the method is to pose your questions and then wait for the answers to surface by themselves.

Who is feeling empty?

Be aware of the arising thoughts.

Who is feeling empty?

Be aware of the arising thoughts.

Listen to the sounds around you.

Listen to your inner voice. Be aware of how you listen and how you pay attention. Do you have a lot of "should" or "shouldn't" thoughts and opinions when you listen to your inner voice?

Listen to the sounds around you.

How are you when you listen?

Listen to your inner voice just like when you listen to the sounds around you. These thoughts put us in bondage. These thoughts put us in suffering. Can we observe how we are looking at ourselves and the external world?

Can we be aware that our suffering starts with our attitude?

Listen to the sounds around you. How do you listen?

Be aware of arising thoughts. Is there a lot of judgement about what should or should not be arising in your thoughts?

Can you be aware when these thoughts arise?

Listen to the sounds around you. Listen to your thoughts.

Can we live beyond the struggles between effort and no effort? Can we have a totally different life? As a matter of fact, we are surrounded by love. We cannot feel and experience love because we are preoccupied with our suffering. What we care for is not love. You cannot call that love.

Do we really know love? Do we really care about what real love is? How can we always demand love but have no idea what love truly is? We are acting with lack and emptiness. We feel so empty. Why can't we feel content? Why do we have so many holes inside? Why do we keep begging for love and demanding love?

We are afraid to lose everything but desire to get everything. We expect sympathy from others. We demand love from others. We don't want to learn how to love ourselves. Instead, we want to get love from the outside. This is why we are feeling empty because we have nothing inside.

We don't have love inside. We are getting emptier and emptier. We always fall into our mind's traps. These traps consume our energy. When you can see your root cause, you can get out of this vicious cycle.

Know Your Anger

Anger expresses itself in many different ways. Sometimes it expresses itself as, "I am angry." Sometimes the anger expresses itself in self-injury or by attacking others. Sometimes anger makes a relationship inharmonious.

For some people, the anger weighs on their life. Some people fight with their partner. Some people repress their anger and become victims themselves. Whatever the consequences might be, they show up as different forms of anger.

If we cannot see our suffering patterns, we will remain stuck with them

Why Your Anger Never Leaves?

Why is your anger always there? What feeds it? If we cannot find the root cause of our anger, anger will express itself in many different ways in our life.

The reason your anger can survive and thrive is because of your thoughts.

Please pay attention to your thoughts as they arise when you are angry. These thoughts and ideas feed your anger. Only when you can see how your belief sets and ideas create your anger can this energy of anger be dissolved.

Anger expresses itself in many different ways. Sometimes we express our anger. Sometimes we repress it. Whether you express it or not, your inner belief set feeds the anger. After a long time, you accumulate a lot of angry energy and become bitter. Accumulated angry energy creates resentment and bitterness.

We have to be aware of our anger patterns. Why are we angry? How do we express our anger? We have to be aware of our anger patterns and know what they are about.

The Importance of Staying Still

What do you do when your angry belief sets get triggered? Our difficulty is that we are easily driven by our thoughts and belief sets. When we are driven by the triggering belief set, we become angry. It's a vicious cycle at work. It's very important to be aware at the moment when the thoughts start to drive us. Be present with your anger.

Before we learned how to let go of our suffering patterns we always tried our best to get rid of the angry feeling or told ourselves that we shouldn't get angry. In doing so, we were creating an "anger bomb" which could explode anytime. The ways we treat our anger provides it with the nourishment to survive.

We don't need to do anything when we are angry. All we need to do is to observe. Be very careful of your every thought associated with your anger. If you can see the belief set beneath your anger, your anger disappears by itself.

Not Allowed and Taken for Granted

If the thought of "this is not allowed" arises, just be with it. Feel it. Don't be driven by it. Be present with your "not allowed." Be with it for a while. Dig deep and be with it. When our energy is not strong enough and we are not still, we will be stuck in this cycle.

If the thought "I work hard and I deserve to get what I deserve" shows up, just release this thought pattern and understand this thought. If you dig deep, you will see that you treat your life like a business deal. If the deal is successful, you get happy; if not, you get grumpy.

Realize the Truth Hidden in Your Anger

Most of the time when you release your anger, you will get stuck at one point and have difficulty to move on from there. You are getting stuck because there is a wound beneath your anger. This wound is so painful and it is stuck in your body, soul, and consciousness.

Please concentrate all of your energy on being present and staying still. Let yourself be totally still. Accept this wound and listen to its message. Be with this injury and let it express itself. Let this injury tell you all of its hardships and pain. You will then understand that we create all of these wounds ourselves. It is because we have expectations about others and we take them for granted. Once they don't meet our demands, we get upset.

What will you see? When you are demanding something in return, when you are implicitly striking a deal; you get upset when the people you help don't appreciate your help.

Suzhen Liu

With the help of The Letting Go Method you will realize that no one created your suffering but you yourself.

Angry at Not Being Loved

If a mother only gives the good stuff to her son and not to her daughter, how will the daughter feel? She will feel unfairly treated and get angry. Why does the mother's behavior upset the daughter? Because the daughter doesn't feel loved.

However, do we feel that we are not loved the moment that we get angry? Mostly not. Why don't we feel it? Why do we only feel angry and have no awareness of the feeling of not being loved, not being accepted and not being cared for? Because we don't know that we need to be loved. Why do we express our feelings of not being loved, accepted and cared for with anger?

We actually use anger as a means for being noticed. We use it as a defense mechanism against not being loved, accepted and cared for. We are angry in order to defend ourselves from being unfairly treated. We also use anger to rationalize the thought that we should be loved. We feel resentment because we are not loved.

Can we be aware that we are angry at the moment when we feel that we are not loved? If you can be present with your response to not being loved, you stop this vicious cycle and your love will surface right away. This love is beyond the mind. This love has no relation to your mental activities.

When you can learn to transform your response the moment that you are triggered, your love will emerge. The energy this transformation creates is huge. This transformative energy will influence your entire family; your parents, as well as your spouse and children. Because you don't mean this love just by words, you express this love with the transformation of pain and suffering. Our mind cannot imagine this love. Only when this love emerges can our relationships with others be harmonious.

Before this love emerges, we are only getting rid of the weeds, without touching the roots. The root cause of suffering is eradicated by the emergence of this love.

Refuse Your Anger, Refuse Love

Anger causes pain. You want to get rid of this negative feeling. However, when you refuse anger, you are also refusing love.

We repeat our suffering because we always want to get rid of it. We never admit that we are suffering. Anger and love are two sides of one coin. When you obsess over getting rid of your suffering, you get rid of the love that you are craving at the same time. So, you suffer even more. Your attitude toward your suffering decides how you will be in the future.

I had a lot of anger when I was young. No matter how much I tried to get rid of it, it was still there. Only when I learned to meditate and release this anger did the anger finally start flowing. I tried to know all my thoughts and managed to be with them one by one. Finally, I felt peaceful and loving. If I had never given myself these learning opportunities, I could never have had experienced peace and freedom.

Our anger is just like a diamond hidden in a rock. You can only transform anger to love by accepting it and facing it.

Understood Anger Disappears Like a Cloud

Be aware of your feelings. Be aware of every feeling you experience in the moment. When you can be present with your feeling and not run away from it, it starts to change. If we can understand our anger and be present with it, then the angry energy will gradually dissolve like a cloud.

We don't understand how to transform our emotions so we carry this negative energy around and undermine our own mental and physical health. The same applies to other sufferings in our life. We have tried to find a way out of these sufferings but however we try, these sufferings stick to us. We cannot help feeling frustrated. We never really try to understand our sufferings. All we do is just give them a label and walk away. Only when we face our issues do we have a chance to deal with them.

Practice Letting Go of Anger

Now let go of the negative energy in the conception vessel.

Now let go of the negative energy in the conception vessel.

Please note that the conception vessel (yin) as noted by the translator plays a major role in Qi energy circulation. It forms a circular entity with the governing vessel. The conception vessel connects the anterior of the body from the pubic area to the mouth.

Now let go of the negative energy in the knees.

Now let go of the negative energy in the knee joints.

Now let go of the negative energy in the conception vessel.

Now let go of the negative energy in the governing vessel.

Now let go of the negative energy in the governing vessel.

Also noted by the translator, the governing vessel (yang) plays a major role as well in the circulation of Qi energy. It forms a circular entity with the conception vessel. The governing vessel connects the tailbone along the midline of the back through the vertebrae to the head.

Relax your shoulders.

Inhale slowly.

Exhale slowly.

Now let go of the negative energy in the governing vessel.

Now let go of the negative energy in the governing vessel.

Relax your shoulders.

Now relax the negative energy in the governing vessel.

Inhale slowly. Exhale slowly.

Now let go of the angry energy.

Now let go of the angry energy.

Inhale slowly. Exhale slowly.

Now let go of the angry energy.

Now let go of the angry energy.

Inhale slowly.

Exhale slowly.

Golden Light

When we have expectations about how things should develop, we will feel disappointed or angry when things don't go our way. We expect to get praise, recognition, and acceptance. If things don't happen accordingly, we feel disappointed.

Now let go of the energy of disappointment.

Now let go of the energy of disappointment.

Inhale slowly.

Exhale slowly.

Now let go of the energy of disappointment.

Now let go of the energy of disappointment.

If what we expect to happen just won't happen, we feel despair in the end.

Now let go of the energy of despair.

Now let go of the energy of despair.

Relax your shoulders.

Inhale slowly.

Now let go of the energy of despair.

Now let go of the energy of despair.

Slightly bend your knees.

Inhale slowly. Exhale slowly.

Now let go of the energy of despair.

Now let go of the energy of despair.

It's a painful journey. You worked so hard and gave it all but things just wouldn't happen the way you wanted them to. You feel frustrated and you feel despair.

Inhale slowly. Exhale slowly.

Now let go of the energy of frustration.

Now let go of the energy of frustration.

Now let go of the energy of frustration.

Inhale slowly. Exhale slowly.

Now let go of the energy of frustration.

Now let go of the negative energy inside your liver and gallbladder.

Now let go of the negative energy inside your liver and gallbladder.

Inhale slowly. Exhale slowly.

Now let go of the negative energy inside your liver and gallbladder.

Inhale slowly. Exhale slowly.

Now let go of the energy of feeling powerless.

Now let go of the energy of feeling powerless.

Relax your shoulders.

Now let go of the energy of feeling powerless.

When we are exasperated, sometimes we develop the impulse to attack or hurt others. We want to hurt others because we are angry with envy. We feel jealous.

Now let go of the jealous energy.

Now let go of the jealous energy.

This jealous energy sometimes drives us to attack others. Sometimes it even drives us to hurt ourselves. This jealous energy keeps us sick and unhappy. If you dig deep into your anger, you will realize that deep down inside you are jealous.

Now let go of the jealous energy.

Relax your shoulders.

Now let go of the jealous energy.

Inhale slowly. Exhale slowly.

Now let go of the jealous energy.

The reason you stay angry is because you rationalize your anger or have a lot of excuses about your anger.

Now let go of the jealous energy.

Now let go of the jealous energy.

The accumulated anger slowly turns itself into resentment and complaints. The resentment energy hurts our own soul and lingers for a long time.

Now let go of the resentment energy.

Inhale slowly. Exhale slowly.

Now let go of the resentment energy.

Relax your shoulders.

Now let go of the resentment energy.

Now let go of the resentment energy.

Now let go of the resentment energy.

This energy will stay in our body. It may stay in our organs; in our brain, or in our joints. Now let's release this negative energy.

Now let go of the negative energy inside your liver and gallbladder.

Now let go of the negative energy inside your spleen and gallbladder.

Now let go of the angry energy.

Now let go of the angry energy.

Now let go of the angry energy.

Now imagine that there is a ray of golden light above your head. This light envelops you from above. It is filled with love and loving energy. This golden light surrounds you with its love and light.

Inhale slowly. Exhale slowly. Slowly inhale this golden light into your body through the Bai Hui acupuncture point, and slowly exhale this golden light from your body. As noted by the translator, the Bai Hui acupuncture point sits on the crown of the head and is the point where the body's yang energy naturally converges.

Inhale slowly and let the golden light flow through your body. Slowly inhale this golden light into your body through the Bai Hui acupuncture point. Let this golden light flow through your body. Now exhale. This golden light surrounds us with love and light

Inhale slowly. Exhale slowly. Inhale slowly. Exhale slowly. Keep breathing until your body is filled with love and golden light.

CHAPTER 4.3

Know Your Expectations

When you have an attitude about how people should treat you, not only are you demanding something of others but at the same time you are pressuring yourself because you will ask yourself to do the same.

In this way, your relationship becomes tense. Every time there is something happening, you will interpret the situation from the viewpoint that you should have been treated or helped in a certain way. You will get upset if the situation doesn't live up to your expectations. Even if everything happens accordingly, you are still upset because you don't think that enough has been done. Whenever you have this attitude, no matter what happens, you are not happy.

Our expectations are born from pain. Our expectations arise because we have been hurt and we don't want to be hurt again. Or they arise because we have been happy before and we want to repeat this happiness. Since our expectations originated from pain, we can imagine what will happen when we have expectations toward our loved ones. Not only can they not meet our expectations, but we also create tension between each other, which only brings more pain.

Is it possible that we don't have any expectations toward our loved ones? It is impossible for us not to have expectations. What we can do is to inquire into our pain. If you are overwhelmed by the pain you feel, perhaps what you can do is to follow each and every trace of pain that you are experiencing whenever it arises.

The only way forward is to calm yourself down and be honest with yourself. Be honest about the expectations you carry around. Admit to yourself that you have expectations toward your loved ones. Admit to yourself that this is the beginning of knowing yourself and inquiring about yourself.

Maybe your pain originates from you having been bullied and despised before. This pain drives you to set expectations for your children, spouse, or other family members. What can you do then? Release the pain of being bullied.

In the process of releasing your pain, in addition to releasing the pain of being bullied, other emotions will also surface. Please release them accordingly. If we cannot be aware of our expectations and pain and release these expectations and pain accordingly they will repeat themselves in the future. Stay alert and be aware with clarity until you truly know the different origins of your pain and then your expectations will dissolve by themselves.

Practice Letting Go of Expectations

Let go of the energy of having expectations.

Let go of the energy of having expectations.

Relax your shoulders.

Be present with the feeling of having expectations.

Let go of the energy of having expectations.

Relax your shoulders.

Let go of the energy of having expectations.

Relax your shoulders.

Be present with your expectations.

Let go of the energy of having expectations.

Let go of the energy of having expectations.

Let go of the energy of having expectations.

Relax your shoulders.

When we have expectations towards our loved ones and things don't go as anticipated, we will feel disappointed.

Let go of the energy of being disappointed.

Relax your shoulders.

Let go of the energy of being disappointed.

When we are disappointed, we feel that we are not seen and not understood. We feel bitter for not being understood.

Let go of the energy of being disappointed.

Relax your shoulders.

When we are disappointed, we feel like we are rejected by our loved ones.

Let go of the disappointed energy.

Relax your shoulders.

When we are disappointed, we feel no one notices our efforts.

Let go of the disappointed energy.

Let go of the energy of having expectations.

Relax the shoulders.

We feel disappointed when our loved ones don't live up to our expectations and then we are worried that they will suffer because of it.

Let go of the energy of worry.

Let go of the energy of worry.

Let go of the energy of worry.

We feel very stressed when we worry.

Let go of the stress of worry.

Let go of the stress of worry.

Relax your shoulders.

Let go of the stress energy.

Let go of the feeling of oppression in your heart.

Relax your shoulders.

Let go of the feeling of oppression in your heart.

Relax your shoulders.

Because of all these worries, we are going to get anxious. We feel powerless at this moment. We don't know what to do.

Let go of the anxious energy.

Let go of the anxious energy.

Relax your shoulders.

You feel helpless because you don't know what to do.

Let go of the helpless energy.

Let go of the helpless energy.

Let go of the feeling of having no one to count on.

Let go of the energy of having no one to count on.

Relax your shoulders.

Let go of the feeling of having no one to count on.

Relax your shoulders.

Let go of the energy of feeling lost and not belonging,

Relax your shoulders.

Let go of the lonely feeling of not belonging.

Relax your shoulders.

Let go of the fear of not belonging.

Relax the shoulders.

Let go of the lost feeling of not belonging.

Let go of the negative energy from your spleen and stomach.

These energies stay in our abdomen.

Let go of the negative energy from your stomach and spleen.

Let go of the negative energy from the uterus.

Let go of the negative energy from the uterus.

Let go of the negative energy from your stomach and spleen.

Let go of the negative energy from your spleen.

Let go of the negative energy from your pancreas.

Relax your shoulders.

Now imagine above your head that there is a ray of golden light. This golden light is full of loving energy. This golden light is radiating the warmth of love.

Now breathe gently. Slowly breathe in this golden light from the Bai Hui acupuncture point. Inhale slowly. Exhale slowly. Let this golden light circulate through your whole body from the conception vessel to the governing vessel.

Once more, slowly breathe in this loving golden light from the Bai Hui point. Let it circulate from the conception vessel to the governing vessel.

Once more, slowly breathe in this loving golden light from the Bai Hui point. Let it circulate from the conception vessel to the governing vessel.

Let this golden light flow through your body as it expands itself from the Bai Hui point.

This golden light flows through your Bai Hui point and expands itself.

This golden light is expanding from your body.

Now send this golden light to your loved one.

Now imagine your loved one is infused with this golden light. Imagine this golden light is above his head. Slowly he is enveloped with this golden light. This golden light is descending upon him from his head to his toes.

Once more, send this golden light to your loved one. Imagine your loved one is standing in front of you. Envelop him with this golden light.

Practice Letting Go of Entanglement Energy

If our inquiry and observation cannot touch our heart and soul, our suffering will stay stuck. If we can understand our suffering only from the mind perspective, our suffering will continue to repeat itself. We will have endless issues waiting to be resolved.

If we can understand our issues from our heart and soul dimension, we dive deep into our consciousness. To purify our soul, the most important thing is to clean and heal the sufferings. To clean our soul, the first thing is to release these sufferings.

Many people have difficulties letting go of the people who once hurt them. Sometimes this entanglement and resentment can be so deeply buried into the sub consciousness of our being that it takes a lot of learning to face this entanglement. We need to purify our soul or this entanglement energy will follow us, even over different lifetimes and steer our soul towards these past connections. Your life experiences and the issues you have to deal with, as well as your learning opportunities all center around these entanglements.

To let go of this entanglement that hugely influences your life and soul, relax your shoulders.

Inhale slowly. Exhale slowly.

Now let go of the people who hurt you. Release the entanglement energy.

Let your mouth move toward your chest.

Now let go of this entanglement energy.

"Now I let go of the energy of the people who hurt me."

Now let go of this entangled energy.

When you release the people who hurt you, if there is a name that comes to mind, just add in the name. "Now release the entangled energy between (name) and me."

Now let go of the people who hurt you. Release the entanglement energy.

Now let go of the entanglement between (name) and you, now release this entangling energy.

Now let go of the energy of the people who hurt you.

If you can remember their names and faces, just add them into your letting go practices.

Now let go of this entanglement energy. Now let go of this entangling energy.

Now imagine that there is a ray of golden light above our heads. Please send this golden light to the person we just released this entangled energy with. Slowly send this golden energy to him.

And then send this golden light to the people we love. This golden light embodies love, peace, and acceptance. Send this golden light to our loved ones.

Now envelop human beings on this earth with this golden light.

Send this golden light to everyone.

Know Your Guilt

If you feel guilty, your life will be influenced in many ways. However, you won't have any idea of this since it functions on a deeper level.

Guilt can express itself by doing too much for your children. Guilt can also express itself by helping people close to you without considering the consequences. Guilt can also express itself by shouldering everything in the family. Guilt is running our life. We can see it everywhere. We need to release our guilt to understand how it functions and then we can get out of its influence. You have to see it for yourself. You have to observe it for yourself.

Observation of Your Guilt

When you start to observe yourself, you can discover your obstacles in everyday life. Once you can see your obstacle, your heart and awareness will become sharp. The more you observe yourself, the sharper you become. Towards the end, whenever you see your obstacle, you can release it automatically. You release your suffering layer by layer, and then you can release bigger and bigger obstacles, or deeper and deeper issues. During this process, don't use your mind. Just observe yourself. Observe your behavior and thoughts. And then you can discover that one thought becomes a train of thoughts, or becomes a theory. If you can be mindful in every aspect of your life, your life will be full of joy and love!

To live with joy and love is not yet the end. Be aware of your thoughts all the time. Be aware of your thoughts and don't say to yourself that what you should or should not do. We learn a lot of "should" from our society. These "should" statements create a lot of conflicts and struggles for us. "I should do this but I don't want to live like this. But I should …"

Be aware of your thoughts when they arise. If you keep telling yourself what you should do, your heart will become dull and slow. When your heart becomes dull and slow, you will lose your awareness, which makes you only able to rely on your mind. In this way, you lose the possibility to liberate yourself from your suffering.

Bleeding Love

"I observed that I will make myself suffer to make my family feel guilty. And then they will care about me. I will get upset if my family doesn't notice my effort and hides from me."

Everyone will hide from you. Why? Because your love is too heavy to bear. Would you accept a person's love if he expressed his love with a bleeding arm and a crying face? No one can accept this kind of bleeding love. No one wants to see other people suffer.

If a child only cared for his mother out of guilt, she wouldn't be happy with his care. If a husband only cared for his wife out of guilt, she wouldn't be happy either. It's meaningless if your care and gratitude toward the other is not from your heart and just there in order to pacify them. Of course, they will feel even more upset if you don't express your gratitude or care.

To give to others without any motivation for getting anything in return is difficult to accomplish. We probably can only find it when a mother gives birth to her baby. It's really uncomfortable when we are suffering. However, please try to ask, "Who is suffering?" Always try to understand your motivation. You will suffer for a long time if your motivation is simply to seek attention.

Look inward. Know your obstacles. Release your suffering and walk on the right path.

Repentance for Gratitude

Repentance is a thinking pattern and suffering that is created by our mind. It's not the truth. When we fall into this mind trap, we will create suffering and take mistakes as truth, and will hence negatively influence our relationships.

When your actions toward others are out of repentance, whatever you do, however hard you work, you won't get recognition for your hard work. It is because what others feel about your actions is not love or help but repentance. Under this situation, no matter how much effort you have made, how much repentance you pay, no one will appreciate you. You will cry out loud and will be full of sadness when you release the repentance energy.

Release the repentance energy. Let the painful energy flow. Let the energy of feeling wronged dissolve and build equal and mutual beneficiary relationships.

Guilt to Get Sympathy

There is motivation behind your guilt. By appearance, you will get sympathy by feeling guilty. In reality though, you want to feel like you belong. You want to feel secure when you feel guilty. Why do we feel guilty? Guilt is created by society to condition its people. It's a condition for the whole society. "I should behave like this but I do that. So, I feel guilty."

You can see from here that guilt is created by your mind too. You can only be accepted by the society when you meet the conditions and recognition standards set up by the society. We can only feel like we belong to a group when we feel accepted by it. On the other hand, we are afraid that we are not accepted by the society. We are afraid that we don't belong to any group and that's why we feel guilty.

For example, children should be good to their parents; daughters-in-law should be good to their in-laws;

subordinates should obey orders from their supervisors; people should help people with a disability, and so forth. These are all examples of the conditions and standards created by society. We will feel guilty if we don't behave accordingly. We feel like we belong to the society when we meet all the standards and get the recognition from others, getting accepted by the society.

We feel guilty because we want to feel like we belong to our society and we need security. If we cannot get out of this conditioning, all our efforts and spiritual practices are in vain. As a matter of fact, whether you meet the standard is up to your consciousness, or the collective consciousness. There are too many "should" and "must" in your mind. Be aware, be observant, be understanding. Don't fall into the loops of your thinking patterns.

Practice Letting Go of Guilt

While releasing guilt energy, you will feel ashamed and you will experience self-blame. You will feel guilty and the need to sacrifice yourself. You cannot forgive yourself and then you will feel angry and feel resentment.

What I said is just a general direction of what you may experience while doing this exercise. There may be other obstacles or past events showing up. If they show up, just stay with these images for a while. Don't set up any goals. Allow all of the obstacles, feelings, or images that arise. Stay present with them for a while. When you are present with these images, you support your own healing with energy.

Go deeper, layer by layer. Don't have any assumption. For example, you may say to yourself, "This is not me. How can I behave like this? I don't want to behave like this." I disagree. Whatever pain or emotions show up, don't resist them. Be present with them. After we inquire to the origin, we will see the real cause, and our soul will get incredible healing and cleansing.

Now let go of the negative energy of eyes, ears, nose, tongue, body and mind.

Now let go of the negative energy of eyes, ears, nose, tongue, body and mind.

Now let go of the negative energy of the conception vessel.

Now let go of the negative energy of the governing vessel.

Now let go of the anxious energy.

Now let go of the guilty energy.

Now let go of the guilty energy.

Now let go of the energy of not being able to forgive yourself.

Now let go of the energy of not being able to forgive yourself.

Now let go of the energy of not being able to forgive yourself.

Now let go of the energy of not being able to forgive yourself.

Now let go of the energy to punish yourself.

Now let go of the energy to torture yourself.

Be present with yourself. Please be present with awareness.

Who punishes himself? Who wants to punish himself?

Now let go of the energy of feeling guilty.

Now let go of the energy of self-sacrifice.

Now let go of the guilt energy.

Who is feeling guilty? Who wants to punish himself?

Now let go of the energy to punish yourself.

Who punishes himself?

Now let go of the energy of "I am not able to get better."

Now let go of the energy of "I am not able to feel happy."

Now let go of the energy of not being allowed to be happy.

Who is feeling guilty?

Where is the guilt coming from? Who feels guilty?

When we are able to see the truth, we will liberate ourselves from the suffering.

Who feels guilty? Who feels guilty?

Inhale slowly. Exhale slowly. Inhale slowly. Exhale slowly. Now inhale from your Bai Hui acupuncture point. Let this energy circulate from the conception vessel to the governing vessel, and release this energy.

Inhale slowly. Exhale slowly.

Who is feeling guilty? Who feels guilty?

Slowly inhale from the Bai Hui acupuncture point.

Inhale slowly. Exhale slowly.

Inhale from the top of your head. Let this energy circulate through your spine and release it from your coccyx.

Inhale slowly. Exhale slowly.

Relax your shoulders.

Who feels guilty? Who cannot forgive himself?

Relax your shoulders.

Inhale slowly. Exhale slowly from your coccyx.

Now imagine that there is a ray of golden light above your head. Slowly inhale this golden light form your Bai Hui acupuncture point. This golden light is full of love.

Inhale slowly. Let this energy circulate through your body and let go of it from the coccyx.

Inhale slowly. Inhale this golden light slowly from your Bai Hui acupuncture point. Let this golden light circulate through your body and release it.

Once more, gently inhale the golden light from your Bai Hui acupuncture point. Circulate it through your body, and release this golden light.

Now imagine that this golden light is above your head, surrounding you and it slowly envelops you with love.

Now send this golden light to anyone who feels guilty. Send this golden light to guilty people. Once more send this golden light to guilty people.

Inhale slowly. Exhale slowly.

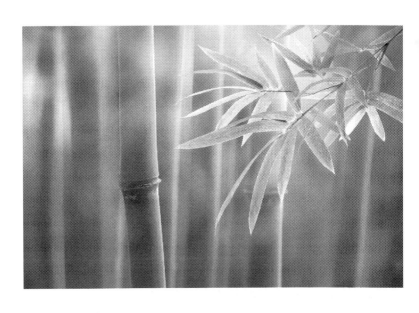

CHAPTER 4.4

Recognition

We are seldom aware that we are seeking recognition from others. As a matter of fact, seeking recognition from others has always been functioning in the background. Seeking recognition from others deeply influences our relationship with others.

To seek recognition is to defend oneself. Why don't you observe yourself if your relationships with others are functioning under this model? If yes, what are we defending?

What we are protecting is image, loneliness, value, self-esteem, fear, survival, safety and among others, confusion. All of these are originating from our concepts. All of these are created by our mind. All of these are created by our culture, education, experiences and memories. We unconsciously fall into this illusion and repeat our suffering.

Whenever our mind starts creating conflicts, obstacles and issues is when we need to be aware of our thoughts, all the time. Whenever our thoughts arise, as soon as we notice that our mind is in action, it stops right away.

How Seeking Recognition Functions in Our Life

How do our minds and concepts function in our life? Under what conditions will we seek recognition? What will we do to seek recognition?

We will care for others or help others to get recognition. If we have no idea that we are helping others in order to seek recognition, we will end up feeling frustrated and angry. Hence, it's very important to know ourselves first. When we don't have awareness and cannot be aware that we are seeking recognition and seeking being seen and accepted, we will often help others with arrogance and even neglect the call if others really do need our help.

We seek recognition by getting better. When do we need to get better? You must have the thought that you were not good enough in the first place if you feel the need to always get better. Whenever we want to improve ourselves, the motivation often originates from having the assumption that, "I am not good. If I can get better, I won't feel small and I will be seen."

We will suffer for decades in the condition of improving ourselves because our ideas and goals are constantly changing. The goals are always getting bigger and better. Hence, we are constantly in a state of not being good enough. We always feel that we cannot get our recognition and we can never feel happy.

Another way to seek recognition is to meet other people's expectations. We seek their recognition by sacrificing ourselves. We try to meet their expectations. We sacrifice our own needs and try to be a good child. Yet, once our tolerance exceeds a certain limit we become rebellious. "I cannot take it anymore. I don't want to do it anymore. I don't care. I am out of here." However, not much later we will get back to our old model of functioning and repeat our suffering.

Mind and Duality

Whenever our fear arises our mind will start creating countless thoughts. If we don't know how to face our fear and learn how to observe our mind, we will keep suffering.

Why can our mind drag us around and create suffering and conflict for us? Because we never learn to face the root cause of our issues. If we learn how to face our fears then the subsequent issues created by our mind will stop as well. Our life can only be different when we learn to understand our fear and how our mind functions. Our life becomes different when we do. We do not need to change anything, or create anything, or work hard for anything.

Whenever our mind is in action, it will create conflict and struggle. For example, we seek to be seen and accepted by the other, so we do a lot of things for her. However, she doesn't even recognize our effort, or worse, she complains that we are not doing a good job and rejects us. Of course, we would feel very frustrated and angry. We take action out of the motivation to be seen but the opposite arises. As long as you are taking action out of the motivation to be seen, you will always need to deal endlessly with different issues.

Illusion

Why does seeking recognition equal self-defense?

It's because when you get the recognition, you will feel like you belong to someone or a group. You feel safe when you belong to a group. Our mind tells us that recognition equals safety. Recognition equals existence and recognition equals happiness. So, we work hard to seek recognition and we think that as long as we work hard we will be accepted. We will be loved and then we will be happy.

Unfortunately, this is a logic created by our mind. It's not the truth. The truth is that you never get recognition and it will never happen. Even if we do something and get the praise, and feel we are recognized, this recognition disappears after 5 seconds, 10 seconds, or one day. We of course will suffer when we are attached to an illusion.

Practice Letting Go of the Energy of Seeking Recognition

The energy to seek recognition goes very deep. When we release the energy to seek recognition, this energy can go deep and stretch over several lifetimes. Please just relax and let it flow whenever these feelings come to the surface.

After releasing the energy to seek recognition we will have much more energy and time to engage in the activities we enjoy, because we don't need to waste our time and energy to seek other people's approval and get stuck in this vicious cycle.

Relax your shoulders.

Now let go of the energy of seeking recognition from others.

Now let go of the energy of seeking recognition from others.

Relax your shoulders.

Now let go of the energy of seeking recognition from others.

Now let go of the energy of self-defense.

Now let go of the energy of seeking defense.

Now let go of the energy of self-defense.

Now let go of the negative energy in your abdomen.

Now let go of the energy of self-defense.

Now let go of the energy of seeking acceptance.

Relax your shoulders.

Now let go of the energy of seeking acceptance.

Now let go of the energy of seeking to be seen.

Relax your shoulders.

Now let go of the energy of seeking love.

Now let go of the energy of seeking acceptance from others.

Relax your shoulders.

Now let go of the sadness in your heart.

Now let go of the sad energy.

Relax your shoulders.

Now let go of the sad energy.

Now let go of the energy of oppression in your heart.

Now let go of the energy of feeling being wronged in your heart.

Now let go of the energy of being wronged.

Now let go of the energy of grievance from self-sacrifice.

Now let go of the energy of grievance from meeting the expectations of others.

Now let go of the grievance energy.

Now let go of the grievance energy of not being accepted.

Relax your shoulders.

Now let go of the grievance energy of not being seen.

Now let go of the energy of grievance.

Now let go of the energy of feeling small.

Now let go of the energy of feeling small.

Now let go of the energy of feeling inadequate and small.

Now let go of the energy of feeling not good enough.

Now let go of the energy of feeling inadequate.

Now let go of the energy of being despised.

Now let go of the energy of being despised.

Relax your shoulders.

Now let go of the negative energy in your lumbar.

Now let go of the energy of feeling despised.

Now let go of the negative energy in your stomach.

Now let go of the negative energy in your lumbar.

Now let go of the energy of being despised.

Relax your shoulders.

Now let go of the energy of being despised.

Now let go of the negative energy in your lumbar.

Now let go of the energy of being despised.

Now let go of the anger of being despised.

Now let go of the anger of being despised.

Relax your shoulders.

Now let go of the negative energy in your spleen.

Now let go of the sadness of being despised.

Now let go of the loneliness of being despised.

Now let go of the loneliness of being despised.

Now let go of the energy of being left alone.

Now let go of the energy of being neglected.

Relax your shoulders.

Now let go of the negative energy in your lungs.

Now let go of the energy of being neglected.

Now let go of the energy of being neglected.

Now let go of the negative energy in your lungs.

Now let go of the energy of being neglected.

Now let go of the energy of being excluded in the family.

Now let go of the excluding energy of other family members.

Now let go of the energy of feeling lost.

Now let go of the energy of feeling lost.

Now let go of the energy of feeling lost.

Now let go of the energy of taking over other people's energy of not being accepted.

Relax your shoulders.

Now let go of the energy of not being recognized.

Recognition-continued

Maybe someone in our family is excluded. We've never seen him. We've never heard about him but he is a part of us.

Now imagine the excluded family member is standing in front of you.

Imagine that he is standing in front of you.

Relax your shoulders.

Inhale slowly. Exhale slowly.

Now imagine the excluded family member is standing in front of you. Imagine that you are standing on top of a stairway and look into his eyes.

Relax your shoulders.

Look into his eyes. Now slowly, walk down the stairway and get closer to him.

Now look into his eyes and say to him, "You are one of us. You are one of us."

One more time, "You are one of us, you belong to us. You are one of us, you belong to us. You are one of us, you belong to us."

Now imagine that there is a ray of golden light above your head. Inhale slowly. Exhale slowly.

We slowly inhale this golden light into us through the Bai Hui acupuncture point. Let it circulate through your body, go through the conception vessel and then the governing vessel.

Slowly inhale this golden light through the Bai Hui acupuncture point. Inhale slowly. Exhale slowly. Inhale this golden light through the Bai Hui acupuncture point; let it circulate from the conception vessel to the governing vessel.

One more time. Exhale slowly. Inhale slowly.

Slowly send this golden light over to your family member's head.

Relax your shoulders and sit quietly for a while.

Loss

'Losing our love,' how do you feel when you see these words? What thoughts arise in you? Are you feeling down? Do you have a heartache? Are you feeling heavy? These feelings arise in you, right? All the pain and all the grief of the past resurfaces. You can see here how easily human beings are influenced by their environment.

Losing our love is an important lesson for everyone. Let's learn about it. If we can learn something about it, it will help our life and our daily activities. It will help us with all of our relationships.

Analysis of Ownership

The key issue for losing our love centers around ownership. How do you feel when you own something? How do you feel when you lose something? To know ownership, we have to know loss and vice versa. When we still "own" something, we have no special feelings about it. When we are beautiful, we don't feel anything special about it either. We can only understand the meaning of loss when we are no longer beautiful.

We feel happy, safe and fortunate when we still have ownership. All of our efforts and hard work is towards owning something. When we own success, we feel respected by others. When we own wealth, we don't need to worry about life. When we own other people's loyalty, we are not worried about betrayal. Have you noticed now how ownership influences your life?

In a word, the happiness, contentment and wellbeing that ownership brings about makes us feel powerful. When we have talents, we feel the power these privileges provide. When we are rich, we feel the power to dominate. When our family, spouse and friends are loyal, we feel that we can control them.

The downside of tasting the ownership of power is that we are scared to lose it. Once we are scared to lose the power, we will try to cling to it. We consume all of our energy when we are worried about losing ownership. It will be difficult for us to liberate ourselves once we are in this state of entitlement.

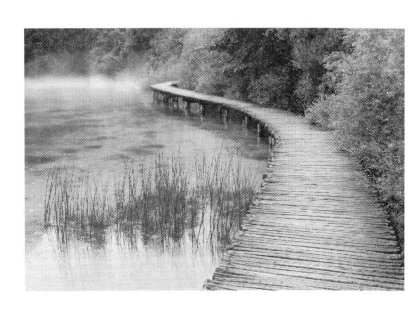

CHAPTER 4.5

Awareness: Freedom from the Vicious Cycle of Suffering

What is awareness? Everyone is talking about awareness but no one really knows what it is. Actually, awareness is a dynamic state.

Since we already know that people will cling when they are scared to lose power, what should we do when we start to grasp? We know our energy will be consumed by this action. How will you feel then? Will you stop? Inquiries like these lead to awareness.

"I realised that I was clinging, but if I hadn't done it, I would have lost ownership. I didn't have a choice. I don't know what else to do. I don't care. I just want to hang on to what I have!"

The cause is that you own the power. The effect is the action and reaction after you have the power. After the cause follows the effect. When we hang onto something desperately our relationship and mood will suffer accordingly. Cause and effect start the vicious cycle. Caught in a mindset of ownership we will eventually lose everything.

If we go and see a doctor when we don't feel well and find out that he doesn't have a license, we will leave his office right away, right? Or would you say, "I don't have a choice, I cannot control myself." Awareness is the mindfulness to walk away from a doctor without a license.

With every obstacle that you are facing, you can choose the vicious cycle of clinging or awareness.

Face Your Reality as Is

"I will stop clinging when I know that I am clinging. But in reality, I still want to cling, I just don't act accordingly."

This is self-repression and self-control. We really don't understand how we are suffering, so how can we release it? When we tell ourselves not to cling, we function under the influence of the mind. When we release and face it, we are connecting with our suffering. When we release the energy of clinging, the energy of fear will surface. When we release them one by one, be present with them, understand them, the energy to cling will dissolve.

Fear is with us constantly. Clinging is just an expression of it. The root cause is fear.

Stillness

"I will lose it if I don't hold on to it." This is fear. Once you are in the cycle of fear, you lose your awareness. To be aware of fear means that you connect with your fear, you know very well how it functions. You are not struggling with the question of whether to grasp or not. You stop immediately once you discover that you are clinging. In this way, there are no struggles.

Stillness is important while you are practicing letting go exercises. With stillness, clarity will arise when we are clinging. When clarity arises, we don't need effort to choose or repress ourselves because we know very well why we are clinging. We don't need to convince ourselves. So, it is important to be present while we are practicing our letting go exercises.

Only you can decide whether you want to function under "cause and consequence" or "awareness." Learn your lesson about clinging. Understand "owning" and spend time to be with these lessons. Awareness naturally arises in you. If you have this attitude that, "I don't have time, just tell me how to do it" then you will keep functioning under "cause and consequence."

There is a beginning and an ending in any "cause and consequence" occurrence. You will lose what you once owned. This is a natural law. How will we feel once our loved one leaves and we feel powerless, joyless, and without security?

Escape

The first reaction we have when we lose our loved ones is pain. The pain of not "owning" any more makes us want to escape. For example, when your lover leaves you behind, you go on a journey in order to forget her. If you go away for 20 days, does it imply that you are still thinking about her for these 20 days? You are merely running away. Can you liberate yourself from the pain of losing your loved one by traveling? Of course not. You may just forget about her temporarily.

Another way to run away from this pain is to bury yourself in work. You work hard to forget about her. However, if you work hard one year to forget about her, it means that you are thinking about her for another year. Why is it so? Imagine it, no matter how hard you work, you still need to go home and take a rest. Whenever you are sitting on the couch, memories will surface, "She was so nice to me! How wonderful it was!" Since you haven't learned how to end this relationship, it will definitely repeat itself again because it has not ended yet.

Someone else may fill her emptiness by eating. She then becomes fat and needs to spend money to lose the fat.

We will find different ways to forget about this pain. However, when you indulge three years in overeating, you are thinking about him for three years. Besides, you create even more issues while you are eating. You eat a lot and you become fat, and then your body suffers. The more you eat, the lonelier you feel.

There are also many ways to escape from your pain; like taking drugs or drinking alcohol, or surfing on the internet, or gossiping. Some use work to drown themselves. Someone uses gossip to forget the pain. Please remember, finding another partner can be a way to escape your pain as well.

The problem is not about what we do but why we do it. Will our pain disappear when we try to escape it? Will we accumulate it even more when we do it this way? If we don't face it, it accumulates in our consciousness. The longer it stays there, the deeper it digs in. Hence, we create a vicious cycle.

What do we try to escape when we lose our loved one? It's hard to clearly express the powerless feeling. We are scared of that empty hole in our heart. We want to run away from it whenever it surfaces. We eat, we work, we travel; however, the fear is taking root deep inside of us.

When we lose our loved one, we feel lonely, empty inside and not accepted. All these feelings originate from fear.

What are you afraid of? You can only face it to know it. You can only become aware of your fear by being with your fear. Whatever your methods of escape are, they are all mind concepts.

Where will awareness lead us? It depends on how far you are in your development. If you can dig deep enough, you will see that you are escaping from a feeling of loneliness, emptiness, and being unfulfilled. You will know that these feelings arise from your thinking. We then understand that we are influenced by our mind.

Connect with Fear

When we don't understand our fear and don't try to learn about it, the root of the fear will reach deeper. Everyone around us will be pulled in by us. When we are soaked in fear, and we don't know how to get away from it. We will influence the people around us. Eventually, everyone will be soaked in the ocean of fear.

So, it is very important and meaningful to keep learning about fear. If one can keep his awareness with clarity, he can influence the people around him. We cannot change the people around us but the interaction between us will be different. At this moment, we can experience love. Before this realization, what we think is love is just a trade and a concept. It's very trivial.

When we can connect with our fear, we can understand it. True love will arise with this understanding. After that, we will not bother our family and friends with our issues anymore. Instead, we are interacting with them with love. At this moment, our family and relationships become harmonious. When you can embrace your fear and learn about it, your actions will no longer be out of the loop of "cause and effect." Instead, your actions become the illumination of love. You experience true happiness when love arises in you.

When you get out of the loop of "cause and effect", there won't be an end to your relationships. You will never lose your power. My family left but my love for them will stay. My love for him stays forever because our relationship doesn't exist in the loop of "cause and effect" anymore. Instead, our relationship stays in the field of awareness. All these negative feelings are transformed. Your love for him won't change even if your loved ones choose to leave. Love arises in awareness.

When true awareness is lacking, we create our suffering by concepts. At the same time, we also create the liberation by concepts. True awareness opens the other door for us. So, it's very meaningful to learn about it for ourselves and others.

The Truth of Losing Ownership

When we lose ownership of happiness or of our loved ones, we feel lonely and helpless. We feel scared. We don't feel like we belong. What do we really lose?

As a matter of fact, we just shift our attention from loneliness and fear to our loved ones when they are around. When we lose these people, we just shift our attention back to fear and loneliness. We are always full of fear and loneliness. It's just that we forgot about our fear and loneliness when we think that we own our loved ones and that they bring us happiness. As a matter of fact, we are the same whether we feel happy or are full of fear. We just fall back to the same empty hole when we lose our ownership. We are in this empty hole from the beginning of our life and we are always in this hole. We only discover that we are always in this empty hole when we lose our ownership. We finally realize that I am stuck in an empty hole.

We experience this pain in our life because we can never see the truth. Why can we not see the truth? Because we are busy grabbing things to help us forget that we are in that empty hole. This is the truth about losing the ownership. The truth is that you don't lose anything or anyone. The truth is that you are always there.

By practicing letting go exercises, we realize that we don't lose anything when we let go of them. As a matter of fact, we get closer to our loved ones when we do so. We become one with them. There is no distance between us. The feeling of their presence is even stronger. This is a love difficult to describe. It's different from the concept of feeling like we lose them if we let go. We feel like they never left. This feeling is even better than when they are still around. This state is even better than when we own them, because we had to deal with other worries and fears when they were still around.

It's so beautiful to let go. You feel eternal at that moment. You are full of gratitude. You are grateful for the care and love he shared with you. This gratitude makes us feel that this is eternal love. You can never really experience this bliss if you are not willing to let go.

We have been accumulating the pain of losing our loved ones from our previous lives. So, we have a lot of fear. And this fear drives us to cling and grab the people around us. We then feel frustrated and struggling.

When we can experience this infinite love without boundaries, the fear will disappear by itself. We will stop clinging to our loved ones.

This infinite love without boundaries opens up a new life for us!

Therefore, the exercise of letting go is not to get anything or achieve anything. Instead, it is there to help us remove the barriers that prevent us from experiencing love.

Letting Go of Losing Ownership

Pay attention to your feeling and response in your heart.

Is it true that we keep losing our loved ones in our lives? Is it true that we accumulate sorrow and grief in our soul with the recurrence of loss in our lives? Are we stuck with sorrow and grief? Why are we stuck, experiencing these incidents and grief over and over again?

Move your mouth toward to your chest.

Please don't leave me alone.

Please don't leave me alone.

Please don't leave me.

Please don't leave me alone, I need you.

Please don't leave me behind, I need you.

Please don't leave me behind.

Please stay, I need you.

Please don't leave me alone, I need you.

Please, please don't leave me alone.

Please don't leave me alone, I need you.

Let go of the energy of being left behind.

Let go of the energy of being left behind.

Let go of the energy of heartache.

Let go of the heartache energy of being left behind.

Let go of the heartache energy of being left behind.

Let go of the person who is leaving you behind.

Let go of the person who is leaving you behind.

Let go of the energy of being abandoned.

Let go of the anger of being abandoned.

Let go of the angry energy of being abandoned.

Let go of the angry energy.

Let go of the angry energy.

Let go of the person who is angry.

Who is angry? Who is angry? Who is angry?

Let go of the person who lost everything.

Let go of the person who lost everything.

Let go of the energy of despair.

Let go of the person who is in despair.

You will never come back. I lost you.

Let go of the person who is in despair.

Let go of the person who is in despair.

Let go of the person who is in despair.

Let go of the energy of losing dependence.

Who lost her dependence? Who is losing her dependence?

Let your palms face each other. Who lost her dependence?

Let go of the helpless person.

Let go of the helpless energy.

Let go of the helpless energy of loneliness.

Let go of the energy of feeling lack and emptiness.

Let go of the energy of feeling lack and emptiness.

Let go of the person who is suffering.

Let go of the person who is suffering.

Let go of the person who is suffering.

Who is suffering?

Let go of the lonely person.

Let go of the person who seeks comfort.

Be with the person who is seeking comfort. Be with the person who is seeking love. Be with the person who is feeling lonely and empty. Be with the person who feels he is nothing. Be with him.

Let go of the empty energy.

Let go of the empty energy.

Be with the person who feels empty. Be with the person who feels empty. Listen to his suffering. Be with the emptiness. Let the emptiness teach you about it. Be with the emptiness. Let the emptiness show you about itself.

Be aware of your rising thoughts. Be aware of your response to these thoughts. Be aware of your response.

Practices to Let Go of Separation

During the process of a releasing exercise, different energies might surface. Whatever surfaces, please don't repress it. Cry out loud if you feel like crying. Then you can release your pain bodies. If you repress them deliberately, this repressed energy will hide in your body and will blow up eventually.

Please stay aware and relax your body.

Now let go of the separation energy.

Now let go of the separation energy.

This is a path for entrance, an entrance to spiritual separation, an entrance for separation.

Now let go of the separation energy.

Now let go of the separation energy.

A person in your life, a relationship, a family member or a loved one may surface in this exercise.

Now let go of the separation energy.

Now let go of the separation energy.

If this separation didn't happen naturally, we might feel regretful. "If this hadn't been this way, this wouldn't have happened." Unnatural separation creates regretful feelings.

Now let go of the regretful energy.

Now let go of the regretful energy.

Stay alert. Inhale slowly.

Now let go of the regretful energy.

Now let go of the energy of self-blaming.

Now let go of the regretful energy.

Now let go of the regretful energy.

Now let go of the regretful energy.

Now let go of the negative energy in the spleen.

Now let go of the negative energy in the pancreas.

Now let go of the negative energy in the spleen.

Inhale slowly.

Now let go of the negative energy in the heart.

Now let go of the negative energy in the left part of your brain.

Inhale slowly.

Relax your shoulders.

Now let go of the separation energy.

Now let go of the separation energy.

Now let go of the feeling of loss after separation.

Now let go of the energy of loss.

Now let go of energy of feeling torn apart.

Inhale slowly.

After we separate from our loved one, sometimes we will have strong feelings of being torn apart or of loss. It feels difficult to let go of them.

Inhale slowly.

Suzhen Liu

Now let go of the energy of feeling torn apart.

Now let go of the energy of feeling it difficult to let go.

Inhale slowly. Exhale slowly.

Now let go of the energy of feeling it hard to let go.

Now let go of the energy of feeling it hard to let go.

Inhale slowly.

Now let go of the energy of feeling it hard to let go.

Inhale slowly.

Now let go of the unbearable energy.

Inhale slowly. Exhale slowly.

Now let go of the unbearable energy.

Imagine the feeling that you can never see this person again. Imagine the feeling of losing this person forever. You can never see her again. You lost her forever.

Now let go of the energy of loss of ownership.

Now let go of the energy of loss.

Inhale slowly. Exhale slowly.

Now let go of the energy of loss.

You feel like being torn apart when you lose someone.

Now let go of the energy of feeling torn apart.

Now let go of the energy of feeling torn apart.

This energy will be stuck in your lungs.

Now let go of the negative energy in the lungs.

Now let go of the negative energy in the lungs.

Breathe slowly.

One more time, let go of the loss energy.

Now let go of the loss energy.

When we lose our loved one, or separate from our loved one, we feel very lonely. We feel lost when lose our loved ones.

Now let go of the lonely energy.

Now let go of this energy of being alone.

Inhale slowly. Exhale slowly.

Now let go of the fear energy of being alone.

When we separate from our loved one, we feel painful. We feel like we are dragging. We feel that a lot of complex pain is running through us. We feel so much pain because we are not aware of these energies running in our system to release it. We feel almost like we are going crazy when these energies are running in our system.

All these energies keep us restless and pass through the pain of separation.

Because these energies keep running in our system and never get released, we are scared of separation. We are scared that we will be lonely. We are scared that we will be alone. We are scared that there is no one we can count on.

Now let go of the fear of being alone.

Now let go of the fear energy of being alone.

Inhale slowly.

Now let go of the fear energy of being alone.

Inhale slowly.

Now let go of the energy of fearing to be alone.

Now imagine your loved one, or family member, standing in front of you. Send your blessings to him.

Imagine that he stands in front of you, and your blessings shower above his head, around him, and envelop him.

Imagine that your love is above his head and envelops him without boundary. Send out your love to him. Shower him with your love starting at his head. Slowly this love envelops him until there is no boundary.

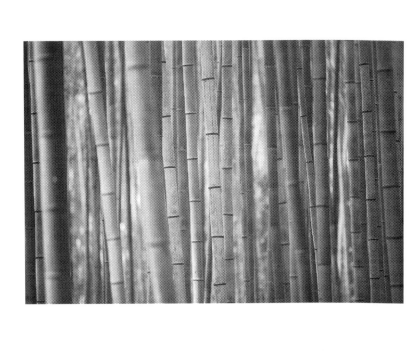

CHAPTER 4.6

Know Your Fear

Pain and obstacles create each other. It's like we have an upset stomach all the time and as we take the medicine we get better. Yet, even afterwards, we still keep creating the causes for another upset stomach. The reason for the upset stomach is that we have too much tea with milk yet we keep drinking tea with milk. Why do we act like that? We are so used to our life and cannot observe ourselves. We take everything for granted.

We cannot be aware of many of our reactions. When we experience pain we say, "I want to improve myself. I want to get better." These thoughts naturally arise in us. We are so used to this reaction. We are so used to this way of living.

We cannot observe ourselves. Hence, we often think that what we are doing is correct and good. This is a key to our suffering. If we cannot observe how we keep creating the causes and dissolve them, we will keep creating more suffering for ourselves.

Anger

When do we feel anger? For example, when we go to a restaurant, if the waitress is not friendly to us, we don't feel respected. If you are a supervisor and your staff talks to you with a loud voice, you don't feel respected either. At this moment, most people will get angry. Anger is the surface emotion. The question is, what is beneath the anger?

We are angry when we don't feel respected. Most of us will work harder to get the respect we desire. If I was going to give a speech, I would try my best to cheer up my audience. If I was a spiritual practitioner, I would try to get enlightened. If I was the boss, I would try to make lots of money. If I was a housewife, I would keep the house spotless. What are the causes behind all these behaviors?

I want to succeed so I work very hard. However, different people have different ideas of what success is. For the housewife, it will be a spotless house. For the spiritual practitioner, it will be enlightenment. For the teacher, it will be an entertaining lecture. We are eager for success so we work hard. What's the purpose of reciting mantras some 500 times? I want to get enlightenment, so enlightenment is success for me.

How do we feel when we fail on the way to success? Some people will get upset. "I spend so much time and work so hard but I cannot make it!" or "I work so hard but I don't get the recognition I deserve."

Anger at Failure

If we work tirelessly to succeed but fail, our first reaction will be anger. "I did it according to your request but you are still not happy with me!" Of course, there is more beneath your anger.

Because of failure, we get angry. And then, we work harder to get success. We can also become sadder, more depressed, and more despairing. Do all these scenarios sound familiar to you?

After anger, you may become critical; because when you are criticizing others, you can't be responsible. "It's not my fault. It's their fault!" You can also become sad and depressed. You can develop self-pity after your anger. "Why do I have such a hard life? I have devoted myself to this family for 20 years. Not even my husband has ever praised me. On top of it, he has multiple lovers."

Self-pity is not the end yet. If we succeed with our effort, we will work even harder and then we will lose again. We feel powerless when we lose. After we feel powerless, we blame others and ourselves.

Success, effort, frustration, a feeling of being powerless, blaming others, putting the blame on ourselves, "I shouldn't have been so lazy. I shouldn't have been so pessimistic." These are all among the thoughts and feelings that bring us back to square one, and you work hard again.

What did you discover during this whole process? Did you discover that you were driven by your thoughts and had no idea what you were doing?

"I want to succeed." You can discover a lot of obstacles in this thinking pattern. We create a desire to succeed.

Many people look successful. However, are they happy? The key is how you feel and not how other people think about you. However, most of our efforts are for others and not for ourselves, enlightenment included.

The problem is why do we work for others? It's because of our desire. We want to succeed. We want to get respect. We want to get respected after becoming enlightened. We feel pain because desire is the root cause of suffering.

All these concepts originate from your thinking. You have no idea how people will think about you. You don't even know much about yourself. We think that we will have a lot of followers if we get enlightened. If I have a lot of followers, I will be happy. All these things just happen inside your head.

When desire arises in you, you set up a goal: I want to become enlightened. So, I initiate a working process: chanting, reciting mantras, worshiping, and meditating. At the same time effort, frustration, and the feeling of being powerless arises.

Fear of Failure

Why do we work so hard to succeed? What are we really doing? Why do we need to succeed? Why do we need to work so hard? The truth is that we are scared of failure.

Because of the fear to fail I cannot allow myself to fail. I have to succeed. I am scared to fail. I am scared to be despised. I am scared that no one will know me. I am scared of being small, so I cannot fail. I have to succeed. Can you recognize it now? This is the fear of losing power.

The problem is that when the fear of losing power arises, we don't know that beneath it is really our desire.

Struggling Desires

What is desire? Although desire is not the real root cause for our suffering, it's still an important one. When our desire arises, we will be driven by it. We are not satisfied. We want to get the feeling of existence and we want to get recognition. All these states are driven by our desire. However, do you really know what desire is?

I feel lack. I feel empty so the desires arise. What is desire exactly?

Because I have desire, I prove myself. This is driven by desire. All the states that arise during your effort to succeed are spinoffs of your desire. Desire is the reason that creates all these states. What is desire anyway?

It's simple. Desire is full of struggles and conflicts.

When we experience struggle and conflicts, if we are not aware, we will be driven into the vicious cycle of effort and feeling powerless. Since we have no idea that desire is full of struggles and conflicts, when we are driven by our desire, all our efforts are creating anger, frustration, a feeling of being powerless, and more effort.

Desire is a state of contradiction in itself.

How will you feel when you finally succeed?

Maybe you will feel very valuable and happy when people salute you. However, this happiness can only last for 5 seconds or 10 minutes. What would happen if you didn't get the salute you expected from others? "Ah, you are not doing so well with your spiritual practice." Just this comment will make you resentful for 3 years. You feel the pain very deeply. You may even hate this person for the rest of your life.

You feel pain whenever you don't get your recognition and appreciation. You will even create more suffering from this pain. This is how contradictory desire is.

You have to suffer a lot, maybe 20 years, before you succeed. However, even after 20 years, you may not feel successful, because you are driven by struggles and conflicts. You cannot bear right fruits with wrong causes. You definitely will still experience the struggle after 20 years.

This is desire. This is struggle and conflict.

Negate Your Desire?

Desire and fear foster each other. The situation will get even worse if you start to negate your desire. Why? Because desire is your reality. To negate the desire originates from your mind. You will only create more issues for yourself when you negate your desires. The key is not to get rid of our desire. The key is to understand what it is. The key is to understand what is beneath this desire. Your desires want to tell you something. She wants her own place. She wants to be understood and to be loved.

If you cannot see through what's beneath your desire, you cannot stop your desires. Who is the one who sees through all this? It's you! All the desires are the same whether you want to have 10 billion dollars or enjoy enlightenment. The nature of desires is the same.

Suzhen Liu

To Be Happy

Is the root cause of our desire to get happiness and stay away from suffering? Everyone wants to be happy and stay away from suffering, so we keep looking for happiness.

You have experienced happiness so you want to keep your happiness. To keep happy is created by our fear of fear. Whenever we want to keep happiness, our desire will arise. And this desire presents itself in different forms over different lifetimes. If we don't understand our desire, this desire will keep resurfacing.

Desire has its own yin and yang. That is, if you just run after your desire, you overindulge. If you distance yourself from your desire, you are repressing it. Either way you will only make your desire stronger.

Disoriented

Whatever we do, we are wrong. We are stuck here. We don't know what to do.

You get a chance to get out of your desire dilemma if you stay with the unknown. When you don't know what to do, the chance arises for you to know your desires. If you say that you want to repeat your happiness or that you don't want your desire, you are fighting against it.

When you admit that you don't know anything about your desire, you get the chance to know her and find liberation.

Liberating from your desire doesn't mean that you don't have desire. Desire can be beautiful. There is always a place for desire in our life.

Since we cannot release the pressure in our head, all the pressure finds its outlet in our desires. These desires become so big that they have to find a way out to release themselves. When all the desires are looking for outlets, conflicts and struggles, and pain arises in us. Desire is the embodiment of struggles and conflicts.

We release our anger, effort and grief energy while we meditate. While we release these energies, we get to know them. In the end, the desire to succeed will settle down by itself. When you are present with your desire, all the conflicts and struggles dissolve.

If you don't know your pain, even when you work very hard, you will still experience frustration.

To Get Rid of Fear is Fear

When we feel lonely and helpless, fear arises. We feel scared whenever we feel that there is no one we can count on. Why do we need to have someone to help us? Why do we need to have someone to count on?

Our mind functions with duality. The opposite side of "I need someone to count on" is "I am not capable enough". We feel scared then. Whenever we feel not accepted, whenever we feel excluded, fear arises in us. However, we have never been able to see that we are scared because we assume that we don't have the capacity to deal with our problems.

When we feel fear, we will try to get rid of fear. For example, if I am very afraid of being penniless in the future, I will become very stingy and care a lot about money. You have fear and you want to get rid of this fear. This is the duality thinking pattern. It's our thinking pattern that creates the fear. If you give up this thinking pattern, you can stop the way you want to get rid of fear.

Alone and helpless is created by our assumption and thinking. Our mind creates an issue, and then it tries to get rid of this issue. This is how our mind creates opposition in its thinking pattern. This thinking pattern keeps creating obstacles in our life. We have to learn to see through this and not to get rid of our fear.

Imagine that there are two robbers breaking into our house. We want to get rid of them. The way fear arises in us is just like robbers breaking into our house. We feel uncertain about the future. We want to have control. We don't feel secure. We feel alone. We may lose our loved ones. We may lose the person we can count on through some separation; some physical or mental injury. No recognition, no hope, and so forth. These are all like robbers breaking into our house. To get rid of them, we hire the head of these robbers. One chief robber can get rid of the two robbers. What a deal! Is this really true? The truth is that we have to deal with an even bigger fear. This is what we have been doing our whole life.

Because we fear the fear, we are willing to give up everything to get the security. We spend every penny to pave the future for our children. Our lover wants to leave us, we sacrifice everything to keep him around. All these issues derive from fear.

We always forget that the truth is, although the head robber can get rid of two robbers for us, he brings in 100 more robbers with him. When we deal with uncertainty, we become dependent and angry. We are afraid to lose our lover. We are afraid to fail. When the reality is different from our expectation, we get angry and scared. We have always been dealing with the wrong target.

If we cannot be aware and understand this state, how can we liberate ourselves from it? If we don't know our issue, how can we feel free and easy?

Understanding Our Issues with Love

How many lovers have we lost in our past lives? How often have we been abandoned and didn't get the recognition that we were looking for? We always live our life under this state of suffering because we do not live our life with love and understanding.

All these pains originate from life itself. It's not just you who feels this pain. It's not just I who feels this pain. This pain exists in everyone.

We can only try to understand our pain with love. We can try to understand the person who lost his lover with love, to understand our uneasiness with love, to understand all our pain with love. We cannot get rid of this state because it exists in our consciousness and body.

The only way we can do it is to understand all our issues and pain with love.

Exercise Letting Go of Fear

Now let go of the negative energy of the pubis.

Now let go of the negative energy of the pubis.

Now let go of the negative energy of the Ilium.

Now let go of the negative energy of the ilium.

Now let go of the negative energy of the ischium.

Now let go of the negative energy of the ischium.

Relax your shoulders.

Now let go of the energy of fear.

Now let go of the energy of fear.

Relax your shoulders.

Now let go of the energy of fear.

Now let go of the energy of being scared and worried.

Now let go of the energy of being scared and worried.

Now let go of the energy of being scared and worried.

Now let go of the negative energy in your lungs.

Now let go of the negative energy in your lungs.

Now let go of the negative energy in the trachea.

Now let go of the negative energy in the trachea.

Now let go of the negative energy in your breasts.

Now let go of the negative energy in your breasts.

Now let go of the negative energy of the liver.

Now let go of the negative energy of the liver.

Now let go of the energy of being scared and worried.

Now let go of the energy of being alone and helpless.

Now let go of the energy of being alone and having no one to count on.

Now let go of the energy of being alone and helpless.

Now let go of the energy of being alone and helpless.

Now let go of the energy of feeling abandoned.

Now let go of the energy of feeling abandoned.

Now let go of the energy of feeling abandoned.

Now let go of the negative energy of the diaphragm.

Relax your shoulders.

Now let go of the negative energy of the diaphragm.

Now let go of the negative energy of the liver.

Now let go of the negative energy of your central nervous system.

Relax your shoulders.

Now let go of the energy of being abandoned.

Now let go of the negative energy of the diaphragm.

Now let go of the energy of feeling abandoned.

Now let go of the energy of being alone and helpless.

Now let go of the negative energy of the liver.

Now let go of the negative energy of the diaphragm.

Relax your shoulders.

Now let go of the energy of feeling lost caused by losing your loved one.

Now let go of the energy of feeling lost.

Now let go of the negative energy of the heart.

Now let go of the energy of having a heartache.

Now let go of the energy of losing a loved one.

Now let go of the energy of feeling lost.

Now let go of the energy of having a heartache.

Now let go of the energy of feeling lost.

Now let go of the lonely feeling of losing a loved one.

Now let go of the energy of feeling alone.

Now let go of the energy of feeling alone and helpless.

Now let go of the energy of having a heartache.

Now let go of the energy of feeling alone and helpless.

Now let go of the energy of having a heartache.

Now let go of the energy of having a heartache.

Relax your shoulders.

Now let go of the angry energy of losing your loved one.

Now let go of the angry energy.

Now let go of the angry energy of losing your loved one.

Now let go of the angry energy.

Now let go of the angry energy of losing your loved one.

Now let go of the lonely and helpless energy caused by losing your loved one.

Now let go of the grief caused by losing your loved one.

Now let go of the grief energy of losing your loved one.

Now let go of the grief caused by losing your loved one.

Now let go of the grief energy of losing the loved one.

Now let go of the grief energy of losing your loved one.

Now let go of the negative energy of the liver.

Relax your shoulders.

Now let go of the negative energy of the pubis.

Now let go of the negative energy of losing your loved one.

Relax your shoulders.

Now let go of the grief energy of losing your loved one.

Now let go of the fear energy taking over from others.

Let's be present with love. Relax your shoulders.

Now let go of the fear energy taking over from others.

Now let go of the fear energy taking over from others.

Now let go of the energy of feeling exhausted and powerless.

Now let go of the energy of feeling exhausted.

Relax your shoulders.

Now let go of the energy of feeling exhausted and powerless.

Inhale slowly. Exhale slowly.

Inhale slowly. Exhale slowly.

Now imagine there is a ray of golden light above your head. This ray of golden light is full of love. This golden light surrounds the top of your head.

Now inhale slowly. Exhale slowly.

Inhale slowly. Exhale slowly.

This golden light is circulating from our Bai Hui acupuncture point; circulating from our conception vessel to the governing vessel.

Inhale slowly. Breathe in this golden light from the Ba Hui acupuncture point, and release it.

Relax your shoulders. Inhale slowly. Inhale this golden light from the Bai Hui acupuncture point. This golden light is circulating through your body from the conception vessel to the governing vessel, and slowly it leaves your body.

Now imagine that your loved one is standing in front of you, with this golden light shower over his head. Slowly, this golden light envelops him and infuses his whole body from his head.

The Practices to Let Go of Loneliness

Now let go of the lacking energy.

Now let go of the beliefs, "I am not worthy" and "I lack energy."

Now let go of the "I am lacking" energy.

Please be present.

Now let go of the lacking energy.

Now let go of the lacking energy.

Now let go of the mindset of "I am not worthy."

Let go of the "I am lacking" energy.

Relax your shoulders. Stay present.

Now let go of the energy of presuming not to be enough.

Now let go of the lonely energy.

Now let go of the lonely energy.

Now let go of the craving energy.

Now let go of the craving energy.

Now let go of the craving energy.

Stay present. Relax your shoulders.

Now let go of the craving energy.

Now let go of the craving energy.

Now let go of the craving energy.

Now let go of the lonely energy.

Now let go of the lonely energy.

Now let go of the empty energy.

Now let go of the empty energy.

Now let go of the energy of feeling empty.

Stay present.

Now let go of the empty energy.

Now let go of the empty energy.

Now let go of the empty energy.

Stay present.

Now let go of the feeling of being empty.

Now let go of the craving energy.

Now let go of the frustrated energy.

Now let go of the frustrated energy.

Now let go of feeling frustrated and powerless.

Now let go of the feeling of powerlessness.

Now let go of the feeling of powerlessness.

Now let go of feeling frustrated.

Now let go of the desperate energy.

Now let go of the oppressing energy in your right atrium.

Now let go of the desperate energy.

Now let go of the oppressing energy in your left atrium.

Stay present.

Relax your shoulders.

Now let go of the feeling of powerless energy.

Now let go of the feeling of powerless energy.

Stay present.

Now let go of the desperate energy.

What scares us is the feeling of not belonging, the feeling of nothing to hold onto.

Now let go of the energy of having nothing to hold onto.

Now let go of the energy of having nothing to hold onto.

Stay present.

Now let go of the fear of not being able to exist.

Now let go of the fear of having nothing to hold onto.

Now let go of the energy of not being able to exist.

Now let go of the energy of not being able to exist.

Stay present.

Relax your shoulders.

Now let go of the fear of not being able to continue to exist.

Inhale slowly. Exhale slowly.

Inhale slowly. Exhale slowly.

Now imagine that there is a ray of golden light above your head. This golden light is filled with love and warmth. This golden light never leaves us alone. We don't need to pursue it or own it. All we need to do is to see that it is always there. We are always sheltered by this golden light. We are always protected by this loving energy. We don't need to pursue it. We don't need to get it because we never lose it.

Relax your shoulders on the back of your chair.

Relax your body.

Relax your shoulders.

Let's be in touch with our loneliness and emptiness. Let's have direct contact with our loneliness.

Let's drop our fear and thinking. Let's just be together with our loneliness and emptiness. We are not in touch with our loneliness and emptiness through ideas and our mind. Whatever thought arises, let's be present with it.

Now let's be present with this feeling of emptiness, not through thinking but being in touch with this feeling directly. Don't be in touch with this empty feeling through thinking. Just be together with it.

Let's be together with our empty and lonely feeling.

It is thinking that feeds the feelings of aloneness, loneliness and emptiness. If not for our thinking and ideas, if not for our intervention of these feelings, they could not exist.

If we can leave our ideas in their own place, then this emptiness and loneliness become nothing.

Without the intervention from these ideas, there is nothing to these feelings of aloneness, loneliness, and emptiness.

So, we have to be aware when the ideas and thoughts arise and feed the feeling of being empty and lonely.

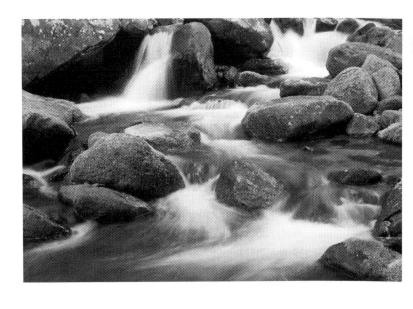

CHAPTER 4.7

Observe Your Attitude

What do you do to be loved, to be seen, and to be recognized? What patterns do we use to get the love we want? What attitudes do we have in our relationships? Does this attitude help us with our relationships or do we alienate each other even more? How does this attitude influence our life? Our attitude is the key. We need to be able to observe how we are dealing with our obstacles.

Suffering, struggles, conflicts and controversy all originate from our desire to be loved. We fall into this trap unconsciously. We try our best to get what we call love, but what is love? Do we really know what love is? Is it possible that we have no idea what love is?

We know that we have a lot of issues and questions and we experience loneliness. We need someone to rely on, to lift us up and to comfort us. This is what we need and we call this love.

We all long for love. We all long for someone to take care of us and accompany us when we feel lost and are lonely. However, whenever we are expecting something from others, what we do is just to drive people away.

Look carefully. Are you repeating this pattern again and again? I can honestly say that most people don't really know what love is.

Suffering, arguments, struggles, controversy; these all originate from our desire to be loved. We are stuck in the suffering and try our best to get love. But, what's love? Do we really know what is love? Is it possible that we have no idea what love is?

We only know that we have a lot of suffering and many issues, and we feel very lonely. We need someone to count on. We want someone to give us comfort or recognition. What we want are all these things and we call this love.

We all want to be loved. We all want someone to care for us when we feel lonely and lost. We want company and we call this love. How will we present ourselves when we demand others to provide all this for us? These demands kill love.

Look carefully. Are you repeating these patterns in your life? As a matter of fact, we don't know love.

Love

So, what is love? Love presents itself when our suffering comes to an end. It is not something from other people. Love is the state of our being.

We think love is from others, so everyone is looking for love and is demanding love. Love is inside of us. Love is not from others. No one can give you love. As long as we can understand our suffering, our issues, our struggles; we will naturally be in a state of harmony, peace, bliss, and at ease. This is love.

Transforming the Feeling of Not Being Loved

What thoughts arise in us when we don't feel loved? How do you feel when you feel that you are not cared for and accepted? Do you feel hard, uncomfortable, and painful? If we don't allow these energies to present themselves and be transformed by us, they will be stuck in our system.

Our feeling of not being loved, not being good enough, of being abandoned, causes a lot of pain inside of us. We can only transform this pain by experiencing it. If we repress these feelings, we will keep accumulating this energy.

By releasing these emotions, we give opportunity to these emotions to present themselves and to be transformed. But, it is key when you practice releasing these energies, that you practice them in a peaceful state. Learn to observe yourself when you are walking or when you are taking any action. Then you can experience what a peaceful state means. Our pain of feeling not being accepted is one form of energy. If we don't give this energy a chance to present itself, this energy will influence us every day. It will consume our energy and keep us from being loved!

Let the pain inside us surface. The reason behind this act is not to vent our pain but to let the energy flow.

We Create Our Own Suffering

Only when we are able to pay attention to our behaviors can we know how many obstacles we have. Under this situation, we know clearly that no one can save us from pain, because we have created this pain ourselves; as a result of self-imposed "should", "thought" and belief sets that we put on ourselves. We think we "should" have a lot of money in our savings account, we "should" feel secure; we "should" be loved, among others. We create our own suffering when our reality doesn't meet these demands that we put on ourselves. We repeatedly create a lot of struggling and suffering. If we always live in this illusion that we can only feel happy after we have achieved some goals and are loved, how can we feel free and fulfilled? Once we realize that these pains are created by our mind, we are free! Know this. Realize this. Your life will start to change!

When we are curious about our pain and want to know it, our fate will start to change at this moment. We don't really need to do anything. When we understand ourselves at this present moment, we let go of our past memories. To understand is to live in the now.

There is big wisdom, observation and discovery in "you don't really need to do anything." It doesn't mean that you refuse to take any action period. When we are in a state of consciousness, we know that we don't need to take any action.

Your Obstacles Are Your Doorway to Freedom

Our response to our obstacles decides our fate. If you want to get rid of your anger and pain, you will stick with it. When you are curious about it and want to know something about it, love arises in you. When love arises in your relationships, your suffering and anger will come to an end.

As a matter of fact, "obstacle" is just a term. We feel that it is an obstacle because we are not aware of its true nature. It only becomes an obstacle when we are influenced by it without any consciousness.

When we are aware of the obstacle's true nature, it transforms into the nutrition that nurtures our growth and development. Anytime we come across any obstacles, if we take the approach to get rid of them, we will get stuck in the same obstacles and repeat the suffering. It's not what happens that causes the suffering, it's our attitude that causes the suffering.

We Are All Well Connected

We are not alone. You are not just yourself. The whole universe exists in each of us. Your children, life partners, parents, classmates, co-workers. You are connected with so many people. You are never alone.

People around you carry their own obstacles and belief sets. When they are suffering, you cannot feel fine. On the contrary, when you are suffering, when you are in pain, they will feel terrible as well. Your pain is not only your pain. So, when you know your obstacles and your patterns, you are not only benefiting yourself. All the people around you will benefit too.

This is why we have to keep learning.

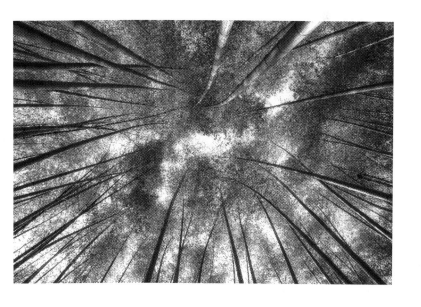

Printed in the United States
By Bookmasters